Blue

Mystical Journey Into Mania

Suzanne V. Brown, Ph.D.

chipmunkapublishing
the mental health publisher

All rights reserved, no part of this publication may be reproduced by any means, electronic, mechanical photocopying, documentary, film or in any other format without prior written permission of the publisher.

>Published by
>Chipmunkapublishing
>PO Box 6872
>Brentwood
>Essex CM13 1ZT
>United Kingdom

http://www.chipmunkapublishing.com

Copyright © Suzanne V. Brown, Ph.D. 2012

Edited by Clare Younger

ISBN 978-1-84991-858-9

Cover Art: "Emerging Lady" by Nancymarie Jones, with permission
Copyright 2000

Chipmunkapublishing gratefully acknowledge the support of Arts Council England.

Suzanne V. Brown, Ph.D.

PROLOGUE TO
BLUE HILLS DIARY:
MYSTICAL JOURNEY INTO MANIA

Life is our spiritual Journey back Home. I have been blessed along the way. The *Blue Hills Diary* was originally created in 1998 after an astounding solitary retreat back to my nurturing source—those Blue Ridge Mountains of Virginia along the Appalachian Trail. The lyrical style of this, my story, was born out of an exceedingly delightful hypomanic episode allowing me to write as my heart and soul inspired me. I was 46 years old when I first wrote this memoir. Today, as I write these words, I am just shy of 60.

As this story unfolds, it reveals deeper and deeper layers of mystical experience. From as far back as I can remember, something greater than me called me to come forth and communicate my findings. The Journey Home is about seeking and finding; and seeking some more. The *Blue Hills Diary* stops short of telling the reader how to find and what is found. The story tells about the seeking and the questions that arise to encourage it.

The *Blue Hills Diary* is written in five parts: each with a number of short vignettes or lyrical prose chapters born out of a prevailing theme. The prevailing themes are based on inspirations from the timeless *I Ching* or Book of Changes, the ancient Chinese oracle. For example, topics include Traveling, Advancement, the Source, Before the End, and so on as initial impressions for the vignette that follows. As I wrote my interpretation of the individual *I Ching* impressions for each of the chapters, I let my soul soar to my very

Source outward and inward and was often amazed at what returned to me to write. During those intense times, which lasted no more than three months, I was simply taking dictation from my higher creative Self connected to the Source.

This story is about Life and how it shapes, sculpts and directs a person; constantly offering the siren's call toward Its desire for completion. My earliest recollections are brought forth from about the age of three or four... a time when I recall witnessing something unworldly and not being able to express it to my parents or friends. As a result, I wondered for years whether I was the only sentient being on earth. In addition, I have experienced something that touches me from lives not actively lived at this time, but remembrances nonetheless. They came bubbling to the surface when I was on my retreat hiking in the mountains those two days. On that same hike, I discovered the magnificent secret of the Universe— animated or not, we are all connected. Everything is necessary and everything is connected. And then there was the Butterfly Tree Island, where there were hundreds of iridescent blue violet butterflies with me on a sunny clear day on an island in the middle of the Tye River, lazing slightly downstream of Half-Moon Bridge. *Blue Hills Diary* is the story of experience, raw experience, and how a few days away from the everyday transported me into transcendental realms of Being.

Since this book was first created, I have undergone many new experiences. Being a Journey, life never stands still. My dear husband, Ed passed away the day before Thanksgiving and two days before our 15th wedding anniversary in 2005. My mentor, Dr.

(hon.) Rhea A. White, who taught me to honor all my life experiences (including the mystical and psychical ones), passed away in February of 2007. Rhea, the founder of the Exceptional Human Experience (EHE) Network provided a safe haven for people who had experienced the odd, the unusual, anomalous and even otherworldly experiences. For her, and later for me who joined her in developing the EHE Network adventure, it was not so much as proving our experiences, but tapping into how our EHEs change our worldview. In addition, after the completion of the earliest drafts of *Blue Hills Diary,* I underwent two extreme manic episodes that left me institutionalized for short 48-72 hour bursts of time and fearful of more episodes. Not sacrificing one drop of life, but rather finally gaining all that life has to offer, I have taken my medicine ever since. At the same time, I began to recover from daily alcoholic self medication binges for they were killing me and have been totally alcohol free since 2003.

Blue Hills Diary is written for those who are keenly connected to Life in all Its levels and manifestations. It is meant to strike a chord and resonate with other sensitive souls who perceive, even intuit the world beyond the common everyday surface. For some of us, it took a few bouts of mental illness to wake up those deeper and wider otherworldly realms. For others, admission was paid by intense suffering or great joy or a sudden shock to the psyche from one or more inexplicable exceptional experience(s). For me, it took all of the above in order to grow, to accept, even honor my experiences of all types and learn to embrace them. This book is dedicated to everyone who has ever sought to find, to re-member and Know their source—it is the story of our re-calling.

I would like to give special thanks to my dear friends and colleagues who read early drafts of this book and actually walked with me during its formation: Nancymarie Jones and her son the author-philosopher Eric Webster first urged me to write about my experiences at Butterfly Tree Island in e-mails. Dick Richardson continues to encourage me to write for the generations to come and to never forget the legacy of Rhea's gift of the EHE Network. An author in his own right, Dick's living legacy as a mystic continues to grow with his personal Knowledge of the unfolding and evolution of the new wise human, *Homo Ensophicus*. I also thank Hillary Dumas for her particular love of this book's lyrical style, including the deeper meanings of the vignettes, and the threads comprising reminiscences of my dear mother. I also am grateful to Dr. Joseph Felser who saw the early archetypal Journey of my story and to Dr. Steven Rosen who encouraged me in sharing the abstract, multidimensional levels of meaning for the reader to decipher.

Blue Hills Diary presages my ascent into a full blown manic phase of manic-depression, or bipolar disorder as it is now called. It is the story of my Life's Journey growing up as the offspring of two caring, yet undiagnosed alcoholic, manic-depressive parents. I am forever grateful for the gift of sensing the world through those larger lenses and not being afraid to intensely experience its deeper meanings and levels of awareness. Something moved me during those days and nights when I wrote this lyrical prose. Something was in need of expression then and it still is today. I was and still am now blessed.

October, 2011.

PART I: SIREN'S OVERTURE

Returning Point

I return again to the source of my inspiration. Once more I hear the calling… stronger this time, more insistent. It was time to repeat my journey and recall ancient memories forgotten, those never lost—merely frozen, crystallized, suspended. I return again to the melting warmth of familiar surroundings and the companionship of familiar places that haunt deeply, echo widely, embrace lightly, yet do not grasp.

How can I explain my returning home to you when I begin this story with my return to home? How do I begin again, begin anew, to tell you about that complex magic—that mysterious alchemy of those other places and times—of what happened there and then?

What has happened to me? I am breathless. I arrive home spellbound, on time, from a different world to tell you my story. Within minutes, I gather a grip on myself and listen to the guidance that cautions careful disclosure. The tension is unbearable. (The muse would reveal her secrets only over the years.) I must tell you now of my journeys and as I do, ecstasy speaks first. Once again, home again with my arms once more around you, my spirit is soaring. I am trembling with passion and singing with song….

I haven't even unpacked my suitcase yet. It's still sitting near the doorway in the family room, waiting like a faithful dog. The cats, of course, are quite curious! To my credit, I did let the dirty clothes out of the bag for a wash as soon as I got home. Then I spent most of the day yesterday simply trying to catch up with the news of the outside world I had left behind. My solitary trek back to the Blue Ridge Mountains of Virginia last week was a godsend. I just knew it was time to revisit those hills once again, and when the opportunity came between projects I grabbed it. For all that has happened during those few days, I feel like the opportunity grabbed me too, and it still hasn't let go! I had the most wonderful time revisiting old familiar haunts and also finally meeting my friend Rita for the first time, after sharing a flurry of correspondence with her.

As it ended up, my vacation struck a perfect balance. Lots of lively discussions and laughter over dinnertimes with my friends that contrasted dramatically with those exceedingly silent times just spent alone with my thoughts in the hills. By day, I meandered around, coasting through the lush lazy splendor of the late summer countryside, simply going where the mood hit me. By night, I had my reveries, recalling haunts from other times, other journeys taken under cover of darkness, being transported once again between the lights of the starry canopy overhead.

Originally, Rita was going to join me for some energetic hiking one day, but as it turned out, she and James found themselves deep in the midst of an unexpected project. So, this so-called glitch in the program became an interesting turn of events. The interruption pushed them into overdrive and they were well geared for the task. I, on the other hand, was seeking rest and relaxation, to downshift for a few days.

In retrospect, it was a gift of time well purchased by us all. While they had the space to complete their project, I had lots of time to wander alone in those Blue Hills again. Whenever I go back to that particular area for a hike or a seminar or whatever, magic happens. This time was no different in that regard. Yet the experience was so much more this time. More than psychic impressions, precognitive dreams, empathic connections with others that always seem to peak for me in the fresh air of those hills. It was more of a remembering—a whole life *déjà vu*—where the pieces of my life, the befores, durings, and afters, seamed together to this singular place and time. And to understand that even *those* pieces recollected are but a single time capsule, recognized as the present life I live; a mere song when compared to the full symphony in which I play, have played, and will play.

Over the years, I have learned that the Virginia Blue Hills are a perpetual source of inspiration for me. By September 1998, I could no longer dismiss their call to return. The siren's overture was growing more and more insistent as time got closer. There was a new act to follow. I felt as if I was being pulled by a magnet. There were forgotten realities to explore. Drawn by both the siren's song and the hills' magnetic pull, I understood, finally, that we were endeavoring to deliver me back to the place of my serenity.

An Aside

Oh, dear, what a strange thing to write, saying that those mountains called me and magnetized me to them. There I go again. The cat once more is out of the bag and acting ditzy. Formal psychology studies notwithstanding, I have heard and read many of these types of so-called kooky statements over my lifetime. Even boldly made some of my own, particularly when discussing paranormal phenomena. But after 46 years on this earth, I suggest that it is a strange world we live in where only a tiny slice of reality is considered real and everything else is considered ditzy and bizarre!

By my estimation as a researcher, millions of folks have had exceptional experiences of many different types that do not conform to mainstream's definition of reality. So then, we are forced to ask the question: Whose definition of reality are we using anyway? In other words, who is the "who" who defines our concept of reality? They? As in "they say" that the world is flat? Or they say that the sun revolves around the earth, or that humans cannot transcend gravity, or the speed of sound, or run a four-minute mile? In retrospect, we discover that these established truths, our sacred notions of reality, speak more to our perceived limitations and fears of the unknown than any valid measure of certainty. Too many explorers have brought home too many tales that no longer fit comfortably with our sacred views of the way things are. In a flash, the way things are become the way things were. And, in that magical flash, we are transformed.

There are many ways to slice up this pie we call reality. While "they" remain, rest assured, nestled safely frozen in time, bounded by layers of protective collective cocoon, I chose once again to return, to question the butterflies of life. While in the Blue Hills, they broke free—and by destiny or free will, I was there this time to dance with them.

Difficult Beginnings

I test again in the world and find myself lacking. The calling returns me ever deeper into my solitude, on a journey I know not where it will eventually lead. In this, beginning again, I struggle to take form while surrendering to the confusion that enfolds and surrounds me.

There is so much I want to share with you about my vacation in the mountains. I already realize that this cannot be written as a linear story, a nice sequencing of events. "I came, I saw, and I conquered" just won't work in this case, although it certainly would be a whole lot easier to write. And even though my primary experience takes place over only a couple of days, nested inside those events are old haunts gathered and new specters gathering. Even today, as I write and revise these words, they continue to live with me. (It appears that I must have brought them home in my suitcase after all!) Those haunts and specters that once upon a time were folded tightly away into the deep recesses of my psyche—my soul—were once again unfolded and released; shaken out to wear once again in their original coat of many colors.

During those few magical days in the Blue Hills, I moved effortlessly backwards and forwards in time, pulled by places of distant memories and drawn to scenes of future glimmerings. As I recall those days again today and retrace those steps, once again, I dance to their music.

Indeed, it didn't have to be this way. I didn't have to tell you my story. It would have been a whole lot easier if I had simply brought back a roll of 10-20 Kodak moment snapshots. You know, those breathtaking "ooohsome" pictures of the local flora and fauna? Those with highlights of adventures ventured, complete with a three-minute narration in whimsical overtones to the tune, "How I spent my late summer vacation?"

Then we could share notes together, comparing superficial features of our vacations. But, what of the depths? Have you ever noticed that when you recall the highlights, the events of an excursion, you are (in truth) actually gathering once again *back inside to yourself* the vivid pictures and pleasures of that trip out of time? In telling your story, you are once again transported back to that place?

While we relay the topical events (just the facts, ma'am) to our audience and show snapshots—the trails hiked, the monuments visited, foods tasted, airline snafus or crowded road conditions—are we not also reliving those very experiences in full motion video? Then we catch ourselves and smile inwardly while we recall and retell those events. We discover at that moment *that each event is magically connected to whole bundles of experiences.* In other words, they convey and return us back to memories of other excursions, feelings felt in similar situations of serenity, exhilaration, nostalgia, and daring-do. New friends met remind us somehow of old friends lost; a museum painting or architecture recalls us to another time with haunting familiarity; and simple meals shared around a wilderness campfire hint at flavors all but forgotten from somewhere.

I think today about all of those "show and tells" in elementary school, sharing scrapbooks packed with blurred photos at evening get-togethers with friends, and my father's two-hour slide show in 1962 of our travels to Arkansas and Disneyland: Stunning pictures, stirring adventures told. Listeners gasp as they try to grasp a piece of the storyteller's enthusiastic recollection, immediately recalling similar tales from their own far-away journeys. In the story-telling and story-listening, we return *vive* vicariously on the wings of explorer trials and triumphs.

    (Recalled stories vividly assembled, calling us to our semblance.)

        (Overlapped ensembles, harmonizing within the deeper intimacies of the surrounding dark, recalling us once again our own close brushes with fate.)
        (Tales of discovery, haunting resemblance to our own.)

Switch back to reverie:

Memories begin to collect as we recollect them, connect them, and spin fragile gossamer webs of our own remembrances. Then, just in time, before we are cast completely adrift in our sea of nostalgia, the house lights switch on. They blind us. In tandem, we too switch on, back once again reclaim a shared reality. Rubbing our eyes sleepily, we quickly escape those unbidden, invasive, now rapidly fading memories. We politely clap our hands as one in appreciation of another adventure told.

But, what of the butterflies that had flickered in and out of remembrance? Once again, they return home to where all memories sleep, stunned and dormant, and caught in the web of suspended animation that rests between the lands of light and shadow. They ask only that we bid them welcome in our reverie and listen deeply to their story.

Their story is our story, and in truth, we return to it again and again until we learn to fly.

Stagnation

I step aside now from my greater remembrances as daily life draws me back into its impasse. My desire to savor pause, to naturally respond to the haunting spirits gathering, grows more distant. Yet, I cannot let them go this time. Too often I have forgotten their promise and sacrificed my integrity.

Still savoring the aftereffects of my trip, (I decided) to call a truce with myself and continue writing these notes before the outside world pulls me back into its grip. At this point of return I feel absolutely compelled to write my story, give it a creative expression. You see, I hope that in some way by chronicling this series of reminders—(to capture) the awesome wonder I feel still residing inside of me—I will gain further insight into those somethings (butterflies) that flit tantalizingly close to the surface, yet somehow just beyond my grasp.

By writing these words, I revisit once more my summer vacation in the Blue Hills of Virginia.

Following

I withdraw from desired outcomes and joyfully follow Nature's silent beckoning. No struggle. I bend as a willow branch who greets her cycles of perpetual seasons. What do I have to lose when I surrender to this ancient wisdom? She replies, and points me on my way.

The basic premise of this story begins with an uncanny sense of being called to return to the Blue Ridge Mountains. The whole story spans only 72 hours and is limited to less than 20 square miles of geography located in Nelson County, Virginia.

How can I describe the indescribable?

I will have to trust that actual events offered in an orderly sequence will prompt recall of the whole experience. The whole experience, in turn, is a result of many individual recollections and associations—those timeless echoes projected onto one background screen called my life. Yet, these projections go beyond my own personal life story to include sight and sound bytes that we all collectively share, experience in some form or another. Those bytes that perpetually haunt us—both pulling us further outside and away from everyday reality and pushing us deeper inside into our remembering place—to our own validation of Knowing.

The events reported are anchored only on a few tangible facts. This story is based on my experience, my truth, my coming to Knowing.

If you are looking for facts and tangible proofs, I can offer few to none. If you are looking for sensational wowees such as apocalyptic prophecies, alien sightings and abductions, magical powers revealed, shaman vision-quests, miraculous apparitions, controlling conspiracies, channeled messages from a master of the universe, or an imminent influx of the body snatchers, I can offer you none.

Instead, I share my own hints and harmonies, undertones and overtones that touch into many of these themes and more of these tales. Each of us must find our own truths, our own way depending on experience, background, and essential nature. My truths are not your truths, we each find our own. The best that I can do is to offer what I have discovered along the way.

Yet, as I write these early paragraphs, I continue to be in awe at the timing and placing of this most recent experience in my life. Finally, beginning to understand and gather wholly from these experiences that there is so much more we share beyond our everyday mechanistic, deterministic, cause-effect perceptions of the world. It is scary to begin this story. In actuality it is rather a leap of faith to share these words with you or anyone at all.

It would be so much easier to just forget the whole situation.

My first lesson of the Journey was to trust, simply trust, that whatever happens *is, has been, and will be* perfect happenings in every way.

Even Rita and James's change of plans was taken in stride. In retrospect on my drive home, I realized that those types of "meaningful interruptions" had allowed me the grace to be on my own in the mountains. I could really soul connect again, recalling that I am safe and protected wherever I go and that my adventuresome spirit is alive and well whenever I listen deeply to whatever calls me.

That labyrinth wilderness experience in retrospect was a communion with Nature. Such feelings of peace and grace; I still feel it today as I write these words. It had been a long time since I had taken the opportunity to be so quiet, at still point with no pushes or pulls externally. I had to physically remove myself, get away from the everyday in order to gain geographical and emotional distance and simply relax. Such is the wisdom of the ages on the benefits of vacation! And I discovered once again that the world can spin on just fine for a few days, without me contributing to the daily grind.

Selecting a beginning to a story—any story—is arbitrary. So, I'll begin by telling my story as the experiences of the trip unfolded for me. Outside of mind meld, this method of storytelling will have to suffice for now!

Assembling

I gather the greetings and good wishes of those who have gone before me on this day. Included are the former me's recalled, remembered as one together. Those parts separated in their various forms are gathered again, assembled from broken bits of facsimiles that have been scattered far and wide over the years.

After a leisurely, although hot and humid, afternoon drive from here to there, I arrived to stay at this little homey roadside motel. My husband Ed and I have stayed there before over the years when we have visited our friend Dianne. Nice owners, friendly and the place always immaculately clean. Good-hearted people too, taking in the stray or hurt cats and dogs that are often left at the roadside nearby and making or finding them homes.

The drive was perfect in its paces. The new car came through with flying colors in her first road test. It had a super stereo with more features than I would ever care to learn except to find the classical music stations and air conditioning that cocooned me in relative (butterfly) comfort while the world outside was quickly blazing into another record hot and sticky day. In fact, I would find that the car throughout the whole metamorphosis experience was wonderful! She drove like a dream and later in the mountains took those tight curves around rock and cliffs like my second hand—responsive as all get out. Guess you could say that this venture was also a bonding experience with my new car! But I am getting ahead of myself again.

Didn't take a nap when I arrived, just showered and enjoyed some quiet time before going to dinner at this great local café. Always enjoy the food at this place! The pace is leisurely; the ambiance friendly and warm. Ordered my favorite—always have that dinner when I visit—spinach and feta cheese pastry and a great garden grown salad. Couldn't eat it all (never can!), but just took my time and savored every bite, sipped a glass of local country wine and stared out the window as the Blue Hills moved through their gradual late summer evening sunset.

When I returned to my room, I called Ed to chat for a bit and then called Rita. She said that they were under the gun with a web site development crunch. We would not be able to get together until the next afternoon. My visit to the Blue Ridge Mountains in Virginia had been planned to include meeting Rita for the first time. Yet we talked like old friends just visiting again. After all, we had been e-mailing and "talked" over that mode quite intensely this past year! It was great to hear her real voice; she sounded just as excited about meeting me in person for the first time as I was to finally be meeting her. She was most apologetic with the change of plans. In retrospect, I think in her wisdom she also knew that this sojourn I was making had less to do with human interaction than it did with—Dear Lord, I hate this phrase—finding myself.

I too had a sense of this already, so the change of plans was no big deal of the cards. I took them in stride, looking forward even more to visiting my magic mountain area in the mornings and mid-days, knowing that we would have fun time together for the afternoons and evenings. This was certainly shaping up to be a real vacation treat! No clock, no books ("forgot" to bring them!), no TV noise, no dinners to plan, no ringing phones, no computer e-mails to get back. Yes, indeed, I was truly on my own time.

Woke up the first morning just before dawn (as always), bolted down two short Styrofoams of coffee, then grabbed a couple of diet colas for the road. Then, pure bliss simply, I let the car lead the way out into the countryside. I had no desire this time to drive into Charlottesville. There was something much more momentous in feeling about this two or three day vacation. It felt like something was literally pulling me back into those hills. It was an offer I could no longer refuse, nor postpone.

I already had an inkling of it, nothing specific and certainly nothing planned in any detail. But during the past several weeks I had felt an ever growing, even uncanny, haunting sense of calling to return to this area of the Virginia Blue Ridge. Over the years this area that had always revived and rejuvenated me—always—as in a 100% probability of a royal flush dealt straight out from the cards. Those ancient hollows with their weathered life-worn hills—called mountains—were connected to me in ways that I could not yet put my finger on. But there was no mistaking that particular quality, that growing urge to return. It was like being simultaneously pushed and pulled toward something unnamed, mixed with a sense of fate, a meeting with destiny.

This alone I did know: it was time to return, refuel, and reconnect.

The Cabin

Although Dianne wasn't at her country home that week, I took the roads to her cabin anyway. Got there just as the sun was barely rising above the lower hills and before the bugs were out in force. What delicious solitude! Nature alone in drowsy reanimation, another new day's promise reflected in humming fluttering breathing sounds, where the only human sounds that morning were echoed throughout the valley-hills in sweet harmonies of distant church bells.

Even though the area on the other side of the hilltop was undergoing construction, Dianne's home had been built several years ago and away from the construction blight and noisy equipment that would surely start up again later that morning. Ed and I had visited Dianne when she had first staked this, her territory, her land, four years earlier. She had been a weekend traveler then, leaving the frantic stockbroker life of the work week to spend working weekends living in a tent, two dogs in tow. In those primitive days, she sustained herself with rations of tuna and campfire soups while she paced these grounds marking her eventual habitat along visionary geometries of potentials for cabin, gardens, beehives and horse pasture.

On this weekday I visited, her rustic three-level cabin sat dormant, silent and unoccupied, along the backtop of one magnificent blue hill. I walked and paced the grounds to see what she had developed over the past two years.

After about fifteen minutes of pacing, wouldn't you know it? I was full of the need to pee. Due to this call of nature and the fact that I was rather reluctant to drive down the mountain to the closest mom-and-pop country relief gas station (rather than gas relief station), I elected to just do what all of the rest of nature does when the urge hits: I peed outside. A first in decades! And my shoes even stayed dry! In that very act of "going" outdoors to relieve nature's call, I felt that I had, in some strange way, reclaimed my own sense of territory within those blue mountains. Then I returned to some sort of (controversial) civilized human behavior—locating a comfortable rod-iron-straight-backed Victorian chair, smoking a cigarette or two and refilling, popping the top off of one of my ubiquitous diet sodas.

The round table and rod chair faced the eastern sun, just as morning was rising through the canopy of endless trees, meeting mountains of hills intersecting as far as I could see. The smoky mist was rising to validate; ground warming upwards to meet the early sun. What had been hazy and foreshadowed even a few moments before was turning into sparkling clarity and vibrant color, presaging the days to come. It seemed to me (for all intents and purposes) to herald (along with the distant church bells echoing in the distance) another incredibly bright, Indian Summer day.

Too, the cadence of bird choruses foretold the theme of the returning day—
              harbingers that warned, in their
      accelerated early activity—
                  of another blazing hot, humid
          day in the Old South.

My eyes began to soften with the rising warmth. Once again I allowed myself to transport, to shift the focus of my natural senses, to step outside the vehicle of my physical body.

> I didn't desire to go very far that morning...
> I was just testing my wings.

Humming along with songs of sound, color, and motion that surround me, I enter into them and begin to blend and merge into the early morning scene.

The skittering brown rabbit foraged dew-soaked garden lettuces that marked the edges between planted, civilized grass and wild, brushy jungle. Thickets were already beginning to teem with strange multi-lensed, winged, anomalous insects (many of which I had never seen the likes of before) that stroked and encouraged sweet nectar from fragrant, milky-thistled wildflowers surrounding. Mourning doves cooed and ladybugs flitted. A racy striped lizard halted mid-stride as he spied on me, all the while shifting alternate feet on the warming gravel, before disappearing once again into larger, warmer rocks below. The bees in the nearby hives were just warming up their buzz to swarm.

A pair of eagles drifted lazily overhead.

In that state of peace and heightened

awareness I said a prayer for this new dawning day—
that the magic of that mountain area speak to me in its
ways so that I would better understand the ties, the
connections and callings that I have repeatedly -over
the course of almost two decades - felt whenever I
visited this area.

I asked for wisdom to understand. What did
this area represent for me? Why did it resonate within
me and at times even haunt me whenever I was away?

Why now was the calling so strong that I
literally dropped everything to be there then?

Why how did I, synchronistically, just in time,
receive the exact funds sorely needed to buy my new
car so I could drive the distance?

Why Now? How Now? I, the patronymic
surnamed Brown asked.

Then I sealed and released my quest with my heart
and soul, and absolutely trusted at that moment to let
Spirit guide me for the days ahead.

Turnabout is fair play.

So with a burst of deep thankfulness for its
natural beauty, harmony and sanctuary, I surrounded
Dianne's cabin and land with a swirl of protective light
before I gathered myself back into myself.

True to my nature, I felt expectant and vastly
contented. I returned to ground, gathered my

bearings, my soda and cigarettes, and then hiked back up the hill to my awaiting car. It was time. Cocooned in my vehicle once again, we drove down the double set of twisty, narrow, switch-back hills and made our way out unto the wide open country road beckoning below.

The Call to the Falls

At the bottom of the hill I automatically turned to go back to the motel room. It had already been quite a distance that I had traveled that morning. But then I, on second thought, re-turned again when I noted that the sun was still rising, only at mid-morning.

(Miles to go before I sleep....
Plus, I wanted very much to locate the Crabtree Falls State Park area again. Distant memory of former visits, plus an inborn magnet for compass direction, and a recalled pioneering spirit
'it's okay, even if you get 'lost' Suzanne, you will be okay'
....led me on my way).

It was a Monday. Very few cars were on those country roads that early morning day. Those drivers who were out passed in a stream of Doppler vehicles waving hi! bye! as I waved bye! hi! back to them. I drove ever deeper into the Blue Hills. I began to search again and tried to locate the source from which they had come.

It is such an informal and friendly area!

This ritual is the same wherever I go, whenever visiting that area. Lots of Appalachian poverty is evident, too. How *do* these people make a living? But the friendliness is always there, ever extended to me while motoring up and down those dusty gravel country roads. Whether the trek has been with my parents and baby sister in a 1964 Rambler driving cross country to find hope in 1967, with my first lover and new husband in the early 1970s to find educational truths, or my (secret) double life throughout the 1980s to find big bucks as well as spiritual solace,

(I return).

For those couple of days in 1998 September, driving my sparkling white Malibu car with NC State plates, I felt intimately connected to the region, even though my car and I must have (read foreigner) emblazoned for all to see in passing. I observed that the local folks were comfortable and much more practical in their choice of vehicles for this mountainous, all weather terrain. They sported dark shades against the sun and mud. Lots of jeeps, all-purpose vans and big-wheeled trucks took the fast track that day as I simply meandered along.

Speed is relative.

In retrospect, I must have stuck out like a sore thumb. To their credit, they waved enthusiastically as they passed and encouraged me all along my travels.

I will forever be grateful.

To my joy, I remembered and easily found the road to the Crabtree Falls Park. Once again that morning, I began to climb. Up again I drove, once more to another steep, twisty, rocky passage of another promising blooming blue hill. I wondered then, as now, just how many times have I taken this particular road before? I do not recall offhand, but probably about ten times in the past fourteen to fifteen years. This time, however, I did not miss the sudden LEFT TURN < into the parking area.

I had missed that turn-off before.

Way cool, I thought to myself as I pulled into the recently asphalted parking lot under the protective shade of overhanging hardwood trees. I saw right > away that there were only two other cars parked on that blacktop. Crabtree Falls was preternaturally suspenseful and peaceful for the time being. Yes, indeed! Evidently, I had discovered that a weekday in mid-month September did not bring out the tourists.

After all, I rationalized, I was *not* your basic tourist. I had a *reason* for my visit.

This time I was called.

It was time to savor every moment of this, my newfound freedom. I took my time in full, delicious measure to slide out of the car, and began to move out. In response, the mountain forests and buzzing wilderness moved in to meet me halfway. Then and there, it was when and where I earnestly hoped to find the reason for my returning.

Haunting Melody

My Mother taught me to walk like an Indian. It was the turn of the decade—the one that would usher in the Love Me generation of the 1960s. Mom would take my young girl hand and lead me safely across the two-lane logging highway that stretched between Canada and Seattle to the other side of the road; whisking us away from our sad bungalow home into the tangled paths where timeless mysteries still lived and flourished. Once on the other side, we would release hands and set foot on the soft, blanketed floor of fragrant pine needles. We would place ourselves in another time and recall forging our way through the masses of sub-tropical rain forest that surrounded us. Dense clusters of shape-shifting fern, grasping blackberry briars, and fragile huckleberry bushes

(growing out of nests of rotting logs)

recycled and encroached our path as we moved silently through the forest toeing our Indian walk.

To our left < we followed the path for several hundred paces as it ran along a massive granite wall that seemed to tower to the sky, one of hundreds in the Pacific Northwest that had been rolled in from an ice age past. Sheered on its western face from a bygone quarrying operation in the early 1930s, it now stood in stony silence. Her sparkling quartz, worn now to deep crevices muted gray from ages of drizzling rains, hosted homes for families,

(eagles circling, above, soaring against those perennially leaden skies).

Along the path, Mom would point out tiny purple violets, pink lady-slippers, jack- in-the-pulpits, and white laces that peeked out from their freshly washed satiny leaves of deep forest green. She would spot a knotted root or a peeling piece of bark and whisper of their natural healing properties when made into bitter teas and soothing poultices. To a young girl not yet in the fifth grade, "to walk like an Indian" haunted me with its distant and yet familiar wisdom. During those precious few mother-daughter sojourns together, she turned those walks into a game we alone shared. I gathered that these lessons were special ones. These ones, transmitted subtly, between us together

(not taught in any primary school).
The trick was to walk silently, softly,
(leading with the toes)
so as not to disturb the natural world around us.

The forests were home for all sorts of protective vegetation, as well as whole populations of animals, birds, and insects. In our little corner of Washington State there were no poisonous snakes or vicious spiders or itchy plants, although we did have to watch out for (the stings of) the nettles. It was safe to meander along the well-trampled deer paths; passageways already blazed between stately sweeps of sweet balsam firs and towering evergreen pines.

She taught me that we were never to forget that *we* were the interlopers. We had invited ourselves (intruders) into their world, into their homes and the least we could do was respect different ways of life and hospitality. It was a game of balance, not only of mastering a different way of walking toe-heel, but of quieting our minds and spirit to harmonize; to demonstrate that we were non-threatening (visitors) in these domains. As we shifted focus from our daily concerns, desires, and human needs, we reassured them and in turn were reassured.

I joyfully joined her in the explorations of the wilderness and took notes deeply into my heart. We would often follow the deer path to the upper levels of Friday Creek.

Several years later, I would laugh when I learned that what is called a creek in the west is what Easterners call a river.

Mom and I would often stop to take a rest on the banks of Friday Creek before returning on our hike home. We would snack on a cheese sandwich, or munch on apples stuffed in our coat pockets, and pick coffee-cans full of wild blackberries and orange salmonberries to take back with us for desserts, homemade jellies and jams.

We would watch in wonder as the migrating salmon returned. Ragged and weary, back from their adventures in the Pacific Ocean, they came in droves (to spawn) where they had once been spawned. Swimming back home again to complete their cycle, they would jump over any obstacles that got in their way and dodge the pools and schools of the more local, shimmering, rainbow trout. Mom and I would smile (inside together) to know that those very salmon we saw (on one day) would soon be passing through the rocky tumbles and wide streams that rushed, split around a tiny center wooded island, and later be rejoined (to connect once again) in our own backyard farther downstream. We knew that once the fish made it back (to our backyard) they were almost home, free from life's arduous journey. There then, there would be, just

        one more downstream mile to go; to the other side, to there
           where the State fish hatchery continuously operated
              —year by year—
              sending   out   new swimming spawn to
                  replenish   the
                cycles, regenerate the
                works.

Memories of my mother and myself in those deep, forested woods still linger from our early days when she herself was still a young girl, full of wonder and music and playfulness. Very soon, within the year, she would begin her own long tumble—falling into an ever-deepening chasm of unrelenting hell from which she could not return.

Tye River

So, as I started to stroll over to the bridge at the Park, one man was just returning from the other side. He had that certain look about him—of someone who had just had a good wilderness break, all space-y smiles. He tossed a short wave to me, then climbed back into his all-purpose vehicle and headed down the mountain. I exchanged a wave back to him and then began retracing the man's footsteps. His steps led directly to the half-moon bridge spanning the Tye River and onto the path that would lead me up to the Falls.

Upon crossing, I stopped halfway, and just sucked the fresh mountain air deeply into my lungs. The river was rather low from the summer drought. Nevertheless, I drank in the surrounding picture-postcard scenic beauty until I had had my fill of the abundant landscape. My raw senses were once again refreshed and refueled, on Mother Nature's (maximum) alert. Stretching alone on that bridge, I warmed up every muscle with that fresh flow of oxygen and raining sunshine. My usually sedentary body (I felt) needed to be prepared for the hike up to at least the first terrace of the trail alongside the Falls.

My eyes lifted to spy the river and its course flowing beneath me. To the east, the rising sun was beginning to illuminate patches of dark swirling eddies and vortices that rose, tumbled, and fell over the numerous rocks and bolder boulders, temporarily frustrating and blocking the river's path. To the west, dazzling light snaked into the rising wasteland, beginning to transform the thicketed trees that had been uprooted and strewn headlong into Falls from above. The deep forest trail beckoned me, onward, over the bridge. That trail (I hiked) was dappled, dabs of sunlight splashing around me in an infinite array of randomly distributed patterns. River breezes gently shuffled through me, vibrating the canopy of trees surrounding. I was alive! and profoundly grateful that I had the strength, the stamina, the healthy body, and the luxury to make this climb. It was (to be) a relatively short climb (this time), but I was grateful for the chance nonetheless.

I had no desire that day to climb any further than the first, lower circuits of the Falls. I sat contentedly on the well-worn overlook rock where many a soul and seat (I assume) had rested over the decades before. The waters rushed, trickled and re-patterned in front and before me, making headway slowly over their own rocks and tumbles. But I had learned over time (from previous encounters with this particularly strenuous hiking trail) that the switch-backs and additional circuits up to the Meadows above would overtax my system

(I had paid more than enough dues already that morning).

Yet the coursing of the river, the sweet bird songs, the gentle breezes that wafted perfumes through the trees and across my damp skin, enlivened me like nothing else that day. I wanted to just sit there forever and sketch the many pictures in front of me. But time was growing short; the flying critters were starting to drone. I started back down the path and passed quickly, across half-moon bridge, eager to rejoin my faithful, awaiting car.

    Yet, before getting into my car (I made another > turn) and walked back towards the river. There was this little path, you see, that ambled alongside the riverside. Well, there was still plenty of time left

        (over) that morning,
            so I decided to follow it (no-time) for a
      few moments and
            take another short break before my
      drive back to the motel.

    As I sat comfortably on one of the deep-seated stones that lined the near shore, I softened my gaze out over the meandering Tye River. Within no time (its dancing), intertwining rippled wavelets began to flash, sparkle, glimmering with the brilliant morning sun. I continued to look farther out. Rocky-tumbled scenes caught my attention and began to shuffle seemingly randomly in front of me. Their collective voices beckoned me look deeper into the river, to direct my gaze beneath the surface of the waters.

    At once—as if upon direction from some secret command—all of the fragments, hopes, dreams, memories, broken promises and promising expectations rose to the surface and came flooding back to me.

       The People I have shared times with here and there,
            The Medicine Wheel we built eleven circuits ago—
                  Before and after
                        the numerous waves of
                        short and long journeys—
All threads and patterns of an intricately, vibrantly colored homespun weave
               I have called my life.

       As I recognize it here now (in retrospect) there was a harmonic resonance drawing me to this quantum field, this mountain area. No mistake, I already had the first inkling of it when the call came in several weeks before. Yet it now seems that this mountain area was again magic, calling

       (like a heavenly blue star) guiding me
   along,

tantalizing, back and forth, up two and back one, almost but not quite, across the strained, buckled belt of the worn, southern Appalachian Ridge.

       (Or I on) my remembrance,
     (Pleading while plaiting) the many strands of braids that fashion Maya,
            (our lost sister—living in the
        land of in-betweens)

illusion, flight of fancy and fantasy,
where I could hope to find my own verse
of salvation.
>
> Maybe this day, I could
> begin to remember.

Contemplation

I hear my calling to task that asks only that I join in deeper communion. I allow myself to be guest again to domains of subtle worlds. Small irregularities of Nature reassure me once more in their greater regularities and constancy. As I view and contemplate, so too am I viewed and contemplated.

As I puffed another drag on my (ultra-light) cigarette, I sat watching as the mists rolled and rose over the river towards the rising sun. The mists shimmered (daylight's ghostly specters), captured by the mid-morning heat and trapped in between the ceaselessly flowing river under our overlooking canopy of trees. As my gaze softened and distanced once again, I began to sweep my eyes across the river to the shore from where I had just returned.

Suddenly, eyes stopped mid-gaze. I caught in my spiraling spy swirls of more localized, vibrating, accelerated activity. Attention now fully captured by the action, I refocused on the direction and purpose of its movement. Dazzlingly reflective in the sunlight—(shimmering) weaves of polished color and dance being performed—their metallic glints flashed out at me.

This vibrant beauty was signaling out (spanning shore to shore) from the center of its rocky little island. That island, in turn, rested squarely in the middle of the (encircling) surrounding Tye River. There and then, for that moment, the little island embraced and served as host to teams of absolutely gorgeous (ultraviolet blue) butterflies. Those sporting butterflies paid me no mind.

Their field of activity that morning was concentrated in congregations surrounding two large pillars of ripe honeysuckle bushes.

    That little island itself was bedrock. It was comprised of smooth weathered stones and debris that had accumulated and collected between larger stones over the years. Somehow (perhaps because of the drought conditions, resulting from significantly lower river levels) a year's worth of leafy growth and sage-brush had rooted and taken form.

                      Innocence
    (In a sense) facing mature Nature's mirror
     at once both fleeting and flowing forever as
      long as this Tye River flowed.
From river bank to river bank, numerous paths of smooth worn stones and sharper jagged rocks led to and from butterfly tree island. They formed a natural bridge construction—one that seemed to continually rise, stone by stone, above the river's lowering water reserves.
    (In a sense) the prototype for nearby half-moon bridge,
          a recent human construction
    that provided a short-cut (for people in a hurry to cross easily)
without the benefit of testing the temperament and disposition of
              the waters below.

    Just this past year, by late summer, the little island had spawned magnificently. Rich spans of broad golden grains, tall waving prongs of Irelandgreen fern, sweet sages and prickly brush had been sprinkled liberally with mixtures of white, red, pink, and purple-blue wildflowers. All of this flora in turn complemented (beautifully) the yellow-orange blooms that re-birthed annually upon the resurrected (seemingly everlasting) twin trees that stood like soldiers, triumphant in the center of the butterfly island, holly-like in their height and circumference, perpetually surrounded by the waters.

But, the Butterflies!!

Ahh, the butterflies...
A whole different spirit entirely.

Hundreds of them (it seemed) captivated me. From within their web of iridescent periwinkle-purple-blue beauty they served up encoded pulses (mirrors) of multifaceted reflections. Each one shimmering with a slightly different colored hue along inherent ultra-frequencies. I watched from my shady spot as they sparkled and grew brighter by the moment in that blazing morning sun.

Safely cocooned on the near shore, I peered out from under my overreaching, protective canopy of trees (being perpetually shuffled by prevailing winds). Those butterflies were teeming with (a sense of) aliveness and unselfconscious purpose—(their wings) reflecting the brilliant sun—shining and flashing in vivid Technicolor their coats of many colors. Dreamlike, at play, I watched them.

(I felt) their call to join them on their island stage.

Foolish me.

But (thank god) that impression lasted only momentarily (in actuality)—merely a flight of fantasy (I reasoned) fed by my own feelings of newfound freedom, vacation independence, the vigorous exertion of that morning's trek. Immediately, upon that realization, I became conscious (again) of time constraints and placed my space-y thoughts back where they belonged. I gathered my belongings around me and stood up once again on the near bank of (reality).

Whew!

That was a close one. It was time to gain some ground between here and there. (Confidentially) however, when I was shifting my seat to stand once again, I did send a silent short wave back to the butterflies: Thank you for your invitation, I will consider it and return tomorrow.

It was time to go.

>Time to get back into my car.
>>People would be visiting soon.

Shifting gears to low (to test automatic drive),

my new car and I zipped ourselves back together down the mountain. Of course, mindful of those diamond-shaped "caution" (switchback) signs posted on the series of downhill slopes, I paid particular attention to those parts of the road marked 'dangerous curves ahead'. But, no mistake. By the time I reached the full-sun valley road below, I was fully engaged (in-gear) and looking forward to meeting Rita later that afternoon. For now, it was time to get some lunch and take a short rest stop back at the little homey motel.

Gradual Progress

I choose to share my world with you—it serves no one to progress alone. To communicate with another stems from mutual traditions we share. Much as a tree knows how to grow imperceptibly, day by day on the mountain, do we also evolve. Only when rooted in our common understanding can we then gradually develop fresh outreaching branches of communion.

I find it interesting, in retrospect, to monitor the development of this diary, especially the descriptions of my inner life portrayed by the different segments. After writing about that first morning's encounter with the butterflies and the wilderness experience in general, I stopped writing for a couple days. Duties called and although frustrated somewhat by their intrusion, I was more than a little relieved to step away from the intensity of that writing and re-evaluate the words already written. I already felt that even in their original draft form, these early writings were getting a little too close to the psyche to share. Some of the plays on words and allusions that had bubbled up from my unconscious mind had already given me considerable pause. Also, my rational mind had a great need to marshal the situation, and I got caught up with trying to interpret and justify these experiences early on.

Yet on the other side of the coin, I have never felt more alive, more *me* than when writing this way— telling my story as I have experienced it. Often in my life I have enjoyed writing creatively and been more or less rewarded for doing so. Certainly it has been personally rewarding, representing a common bright thread throughout my life, even if most of those early attempts of expression ended up in stacks of file folders and in cabinets. But this series of diary segments as they unfolded and evolved felt different. Instead of glossing over them to make a nice story, I decided to give them free rein, to just let them lead. In effect, I invited the creative muse calling me to express herself fully, come what may.

I have always had difficulties expressing myself in a linear fashion, although I can and often do when writing research and academic reports. But the world I live in is multileveled and holographic, felt first as an impression with crossed synesthetic senses and interconnected, often moving patterns, which must then be translated into their various prisms of reality in order to communicate them to others.

It can be lonely, although I certainly am not alone in this way of apprehending the world. Others have discovered their own creativity in all of its myriad forms, from the creative arts of painting, music and dance, to writing poetry, science fiction and literature. There are so many ways to convey the vibrancy and movement of these other worlds. I often wonder today where my path would have turned, had I stayed with playing the violin or been encouraged with my beginner pottery and sculpture attempts or early sketches and coloring. But our society is one that overwhelmingly prefers a linear, rational, if not totally logical, way of expression as a common communicative form.

But I read. I read everything that I can and in that reading I actively place myself in the author's head. A form of empathetic connection with another that has shown me over the years that when I suspend my own prejudices and boundaries, the results are richly rewarding. Certainly it is fun to visit other times and locales as visualized in the mind of the writer. Yet at times, my reading is very deliberate and slow going. It is difficult for me to grasp and anchor certain technical concepts or understand complicated relationships. But I keep trying.

(In my graduate university years a psychologist colleague was developing a new test for dyslexia. I won the title of "profoundly dyslexic" with flying colors at the ripe old age of 25). There have been many times in my life when I have had to read and reread, or ask again and again, until a concept or a relationship jelled (particularly right-left, for which I have no innate comprehension and which I had to develop a mnemonic for very early on, one that I still use today).

This inability to comprehend the way that "normal" people experience life? It was something to hide. And in 1998, when I was 46, it was a source of personal shame and still a challenge. To catch the world as others perceived it was a form of survival for me. So I excelled in scholarship and attempted to grasp difficult concepts offered by others so that I could learn the ways of the world in their way.

But the world as I experience it is vibrant, dynamic, constantly moving along many seen and unseen dimensions. It is synchronistic, totally interrelated and not anchored in traditional notions of time (before/after), place (here/there), orientation in space (above/below), or personal boundaries (I/Thou, without/within). In fact, my mode of operation is often considered backwards. This can be read as backwards logic from synthetic thinking to analytic; or backwards, as in how Western society looks down upon indigenous peoples and their cultures. Either way, I have learned to trust my own intuition and know that I am not alone.

With the writing and evolvement of these segments of The *Blue Hill Diary* (and they are ongoing), I turn the tables. Instead of fitting myself into your world, I invite you, the reader, to share mine. I ask that you suspend your own prejudices and boundaries and come into my head, experience the world as I do: backwards, forwards, and inside out. Playing with words and meanings, and mindful of the concepts that we share and those that haunt us as human beings, I play with you. You decide, in this game of Red Rover, Red Rover, whether you want to come over. We live in a wonderful, multifaceted world. I would like to share it with you using the only art form I have available to me today—my painting of words.

Artist Musings

The call to visit butterfly-tree island that day was powerful, compelling. As I sat anchored to my rock on the near shore and watched the scene unfolding before me, I felt a most incredible urge to draw, sketch, paint the beauty. Somehow (I needed) to capture that dynamic place, that scene; to hold the eternal moment in a snapshot prism of time.

Phasing in and out, those pulses of silvery shadow and golden light dappled continued to play on the opposite shore where I had been but moments before. (Mere whispers) becoming yet again, in turn, overshadowed by the brilliant, blinding sun that poured swept through the center of butterfly tree island from east to west. As its approach signaled mid-day, the summit of the sun faced fully on that little rocky island. It warmed and energized the surrounding Tye waters. The previously still, dormant rocks and lead-gray boulders had seemed (then) remarkably alive, scattered throughout amidst the low gurgling (purring sounds) and sparkling (rainbow hues) of the river's course that day.

To embrace, to forever hold that moment—to be intimately connected with the teeming (harmony) of the iridescent blues, sulfur yellows, ultra whites of the butterflies; the tiny pure oranges of the honeysuckle flowers; the brighter kelly-green ferns superimposed upon the darker stately evergreens and hardwoods in the background; eggshell (fragile) blue skies; and dots and dashes of (more seeded) red, pink, purple-violet wildflowers than I have ever seen sprinkled along the ground. Yet, surprisingly, no bird songs (I recall hearing) calling, even at a distance from the shores.

I vowed (at that time) to the experience, to the butterflies, the river, rocks, trees, and tiny minnows in the pools that surrounded me, that I would be back the next day to take notes with pencil and paper.

Woman Talk

It was wonderful to meet with Rita and James that afternoon at their beautiful home full of cultural antiquities and feelings of sanctuary. By late afternoon, Rita and I took a rest stop, then, in the early evening, resumed our meeting at that little local café, and continued our talk non-stop. A light dinner for me again. There we were, like old friends chatting in that café—face to face—we joked and laughed a lot.

Amazing, that meeting. For both of us, our trains of thought would go in a hundred directions at once, yet converge fully on track as we each shared similar insights and stories more often than not filled-in by the other, telling a similar story or remarkable connection. We had met via a precious mutual friend (a.k.a. Feather Moon) and had emailed back and forth for several months. But I don't think either one of us was prepared for the rush of energy that manifested in smiles, laughter, and the fire of talking non-stop between us. That in itself became the joke, and being silly and serious at the same time was the order of the day. Luckily, we had the whole smoking section to ourselves and a sweet, infinitely patient server. Rita, a healthy woman who no longer smoked, was gracious as she recalled former days of a good smoke shared between friends.

There had been many peaceful times between

her and extended family of friends over tobacco, over the times before. Many of these friends of family came to settle. They had staked their claims on the land to mark territories and ways of life that continue to thrive on the Blue Ridge Mountains.

Hearing her story and tying it to those stories that continue to haunt me, they all began to converge. My own musings, always circles of recollections, recalling, recycling me back to those calling fields that rested deep within the crystalline Blue Hills. We also shared experiences recounted by our larger family, many already living on the mountain. Retold also stories without names, offered by weekend warriors already in need of a new way of life; those who chose instead to visit, on occasion, armed with full quivers of questions.

> Our conversations were electric, sparked with sharing ancient philosophies and the perennial varieties of ways and turns.
> It felt familiar.
> We were comfortable in our peace, amidst the smoke, smoked trout and other local field and stream catches of the day.
> It had been a good day.
> For both of us, we spun our woman talk and gathered the significance of this evening tea time together.
> Time squared

as we continued to weave patterns of mutual insights and oversights; coloring our experiences against the background of another long lingering golden Indian summer's day.

Mainly woman talk, yes. I wanted to know more about my roots, the ancestors, the families from which we grew, those who called from distant times and places. It was already late summer, a turning of the yellow leaf, and we well understood the significance of the times. We shared our views of the fates, as told by the starry constellations above and acted out on the stage of humanity below. We reflected on a mutual harmony strummed by the silver feathers of the moon over ages. Gradually, we talked ourselves right out of the door and said our good-nights. Another golden sunset began to nestle and sleep, weary from the day. And the sliver of silver moon soon dissolved once again into the indigo shadows of the distant Blue Hills.

Haunting Melody

Before we moved to our bungalow home on the mainland (where the river ran through our backyard and the fish hatchery recycled downstream), we lived in a small town on emerald green Fidalgo Island. Boats and ferries and one bridge were the only way to connect us to the mainland of the lower 48 United States. In the 1950s my parents had followed their newlywed American dream of a house, a boat, and baby makes three. They were hoping for four, five, and six. After six more years of trial and error my baby sister made four. She was a miracle baby by all accounts. But by then the dream was already beginning to fade.

Fidalgo Island is one of the scores of greater and lesser San Juan Islands, situated in the farthest northwest corner of the United States before Alaska became the 49th state. It is a natural sub-tropical paradise with flourishing, lush evergreen forests which were continuously weathered, watered and warmed by the prevailing ocean and wind currents entering the Strait of Juan de Fuca. In those days, and probably still today, the local inhabitants were connected by a single drawbridge to the mainland. It was a largely contained and isolated life for those of us living there, a small town whose industries highlighted logging, fish canning and oil refinement. My father became the chief "first-aid" man for one of the oil refineries for a few years. This job followed a few years of implementing and then overseeing the first x-ray and pathology labs at the greater regional Anacortes hospital of approximately 100 beds.

My baby sister was born in that very hospital.

I was born in the northwest corner of Oregon, in a little hamlet just outside of Portland where my dad was then a local deputy sheriff. He first heard of my birth announcement, unexpected and almost two weeks past due arrival, over the police radio shortly after 2:34 on a late January night.

"Mr. Brown, congratulations!" the dispatcher's voice crackled and broke in over the radio for all on night watch to hear that night, "you have a healthy, beautiful baby daughter."

My father's reply was meticulously recorded in my baby book soon thereafter, "A girl? That's silly."

I never got the chance to ask him what he meant by that. But over the years I was his special girl-son, his confidant, his student, eager to excel and learn the ways of the man's preferred and valued worlds of science, business, philosophy, taking risks and chess strategies.

On the other hand, Mom would share with me, over the rest of her abbreviated life, that my birthing was the most wondrous moment of *her* life. She said that she felt visited by God at that very moment of extreme pain—had gasped and grasped all that was sacred in life in one flash of ecstatic joy and fulfillment.

Other than the hopeful anticipation and birthing moments when my sister was born, God did not seem to pay her too many visits.

After my sister was born in 1958, Mom finally quit her day job as a medical laboratory specialist and doctor's assistant. We would take leisurely strolls down to the ferry docks to watch the comings and goings of the ferries, the loading and unloading of cars. Visitors needing a one way or round trip off the island to Canada would line up at the ferry boat docks each day. This show was more entertaining than a Sunday matinee rerun of Disney's *Shaggy Dog* or Cecile B. de Mille's *Ten Commandments*. We would buy a fifteen cent box of freshly popped popcorn—with real butter—from the dock vendor, and then bump my sister's baby buggy along the narrow strip of rocky granite, agate and barnacle beach till we found a place to set up camp for the afternoon. Surrounded by salty clusters of seaweed strands, ballooned kelp, and tangled sticks of driftwood accented with tiny black mussel shells, we would spread out Dad's old army blanket and perch for a couple of hours, toss popcorn at the circling gulls, and gaze far out over the billowing sea.

Those always seemed to be sunny days for us in the Pacific Northwest. We would shield our eyes against the pouring overhead sun and the ocean's mirrored reflections.

Mom invented a game: Who would be the first to catch the distant spot on the horizon coming from behind Orcas Island, signaling the next approaching ferry? Extra points were awarded for spotting a whale pod or school of flying fish.

While we were playing our child's game, a solitary totem pole stood silent nearby. It was ageless and mute, magnificent, in its towering Thunderbird

silence. Freshly painted by the local native tribe, it was returned each summer once again to its original hues of sienna rust, burnt umber, cobalt blue and yellow ochre. Thunderbird's eyes were shielded-under ridges, unfathomable, stern—and painted blackest black. It seemed to be watching over us while we watched out for the next ferry. When we strolled by that totem pole, in our own comings and goings along the beach, I would always give "him" a pat for good luck. I would stretch each visiting day to see how far I could reach up its side.
(I was in an enormous hurry to grow up.)

Over four summers of primary school I managed to reach on tip-toe midway up its towering height. There was still a lot of room for improvement, but I was making progress! At those times of stretching and measuring, I could feel Thunderbird smiling.

Daddy had a boat called the *Eight-Ball*. The family, us three—and later four—would take weekend jaunts to the other islands. (I still recall hearing that because some of those islands were so remote and densely forested, homesteading was encouraged.) We'd pack a picnic basket full of Bean and Bacon (a.k.a. Boat) soup, home-made Dungeness crab salad, cheese sandwiches and marshmallows. We would hop from island to island. Then when we were stuffed from lunch and had been rocked enough by sea tides, Dad and I would drop anchor and fishing lines at one or another of the numerous coves. At dusk we would call it a day, motor up into one of various island inlets, secure the boat to a strong tree and pitch our tent for the night. Locating sticks for marshmallow skewers and collecting driftwood for the open campfire was my job. Our faces would glow and strobe in the firelight—taking on all kinds of phantasmagoric expressions—as Dad would tell another one of his wonderful stories. His mysteries and riddles were my favorites. But the one that stands out most in my mind as I write these words today was his telling of the *Monkey's Paw*.

"Be careful what you wish for," he warned, "because you never know just how your wishes mirror back to you."

Artist Musings

As I drifted off to sleep near the embers of those still warm campfires, I could hear the familiar song of mermaids. Their sweet melodies called me once again from just around the next rocky cove. On those rare summer nights, when I was allowed to sleep out under the deepening canopy of stars, I could literally *see* their silvery songs wrap and surround our emerald green island camp.

Vibrant colors swooped and gathered
becoming swirls of robust reds and pulsing purples
that in turn created, mixed and blended into
iridescent ultra-violet blue green sparkles
swimming, spiraling and dancing over my head.
Together as one, in wordless communication, we remembered.

Our universal code of color and sound exchanged, signaling briefly transmissions sent as bursts, bundles of inquiry and acknowledgment (*inq-ack*ing) through background voids filled with no more noise than the deepest reaches of inky, starry nights. As I drifted in and out of this, my Doppler sleep, I could still hear my parents' muffled laughter coming from inside their tent.

Ancient Melodies

Sometime between here and there, I recall standing alone on a rocky outcropping, a shelf of sacred stone rising above the wooded glens and denser forests that surrounded and protected our family of people. From my vantage point, I gaze out far over the forests to other hills rising on the distant horizons of my vision. With language of fire and smoke at the precision pre-dawns of each silent powerful moon, I signal our clan's status.

Billows of smoke, born of wood and fire, sent and received across tops of neighboring hills surrounding, both seen and unseen. At those moments, once again the sun and moon dance in unison, as one, switching places on the horizon of the eastern sky. Rising and falling in rhythms of their own mysterious coupling, their pivotal cycles once again greet each other and float for just a breath above the deep forests and rocky hills as far as our collective eyes of smoke can see.

> Together at once, we all breathe as one, in unison—
> dancing lights, forests, rocks, hills, and those of us standing upon hilltops,
> both seen and unseen.
> And at that magical pivotal breath, the gateways
> between
> the worlds are opened, exchanged, and reversed.

At those places, in those times, I recalled when
>   neither smokes nor wooded fires were necessary to communicate.

Exchanges then silent, totally *unseen* and yet known and remembered—
>   following rhythms of a dance we all know *is*,
>> would *become*, had always *been*.

A song perpetually playing a tune of our own remembering
>   once again the infinite worlds, pregnant of possibilities,
>> mysteriously grasped once more upon those magical
>>> transitional moments of breath.

Artist Musings

Those overnight family journeys on Dad's motor boat *Eight Ball* were magical. We would set camp on different islands, at different times, somewhere within the Strait of Juan de Fuca, San Juan Islands, Pacific Northwest, USA. There and then we would set camp and shift gears to idle, away from the stresses of 1950s daily life. Each of us had our own stresses in those days—Dad trying to make a living for all of us, Mom trying to live in a world that did not accept more from a genius woman than being a genetic brood hen, and me—I was just trying to understand life.

When I saw colors as swirling sounds smells tastes, and rhythms that moved me,
> creating and dissolving,
>> blending
>>> depending
>>>> on the island we visited and my age of inquiry,

I felt that I was being touched by mermaids and whales, flowers and rocks, agates and seaweed, seagulls, butterflies, and toasted-to-perfection marshmallows.

On those visits when Thunderbird would encourage me and smile on my "stretching to be a grown-up" check points, his black eyes flashed brilliantly for just a moment
> in-between,
>> when no one else could catch him
>>> —no one was looking—
>>>> but me.

I tried to explain,
> but each time I tried,
>> no matter how I tried,
>>> something was lost in the
>> translation.

My parents somehow seemed to understand this, but told me no one else would. They said: Silence is a good thing when speaking of things best not spoken of.

I think that they understood, because my sister, Kathryn, arrived as a miracle. Another girl child ("a girl, that's silly!"), Kathryn was born wholly and beautifully six days short of my own birthing anniversary day, six years between us. After losses of babies not born to breathe even one breath, my parents saw that she was truly a gift sent by God. Her birth and thriving came just in-between the times of hope and hopeless—a wholly embodied proof for them in 1958 that all was right with the world again.

At first, it is those simple things we remember—the parts, the fragments, similar to what is left after waking out of a dream. For me, it was gathering driftwood sticks for cooking over an open campfire, siphoning water at running creeks for drinking (just over the rocks in the bubbles), bathing in the island lakes or salty inlets, and ducking into the forested wilderness when nature called. And each time, each fragment would spark a flame of remembering other times and places.

Then, thirty-forty some years later when I visited the Blue Hills again, the scene, settings, the play and the players (both seen and unseen) would spark—

some drift would come back to me—something

more than one child-life of memories.

Moreover, recollected remembering,

the in-betweens, the times before and after.

Calls that continued to haunt—fragments left unresolved—

those timeless and ancient memories,

how quickly they

turn to ash in our forgetting.

An Aside

As children, our world incorporates a small circle of adults whose roles are to guide us into becoming proper social creatures. My parents' job, as parents, was to help me differentiate between the worlds—dividing seen from unseen—so that there would no longer be any in-between, just facts and clear-cut answers. Silence promotes forgetting when remembering, and soon we forget to remember. And then one day we just simply forget.

As parents, Bob and Carol endeavored and believed that they could somehow protect me and offer shortcuts navigating the traumas and painful lessons of life. Those were my early years, when theirs were joyful and they still believed in the sacred promise of a better life stretching endlessly before them. But in their forgetting, they fell. Life became a struggle for them, no longer glorious everlasting, filled with joy. Their fires of hope and dreams died, excruciatingly, slowly, until the final glowing embers dissolved into cold ash. Since ash cannot kindle a fire, they lost their way. They too, as their parents before them, forgot how to remember the wonder in-between both seen and unseen. And in doing so, we the children take note and begin the walk of our adult sleeping, and over time, begin to forget, cocoon and turn to ash too.

Night Vision

It was only a mile or two drive back to the motel after my dinner at the country café with Rita. The evening stars were just beginning their knightly protective canopy as another lingering Indian sun-summer-set and a mere watery crescent of a new sliver of moon was rising. Being a weekday, there were only a few travelers staying at the motel. The parking lot had already diminished over the busy weekend. I trusted that it would fill overnight (once again) with truckers moving through their longer recycling transits, and later over the weekend, offering a respite for fresh droves of sight-seeing tourists who were just passing through.

The night was still young when I arrived. It called me to connect once again in the fields behind the family-owned motel. I had walked (those fields) in daylight at times before with Ed, but now had to make my own way (alone this time) into the darkness, with only the lights of the starry canopy and moon sliver winking overhead.

I dropped my doggie bag of dinner leftovers (forgotten what it was by now) onto the counter near the wash basin and grabbed a fresh pack of cigarettes. Walking between the shadows of country darkness, I found my way back to the back field outside. Gradually, my eyes adjusted to the enveloping dimness and watched as I bypassed the coke and ice machines, (silently moving) over the blacktop pavement until I set foot on rich soil once again. As I crept along, the fragrances of freshly mowed grasses, newly turned earth, and wafting wisteria reached out, entwined, and comforted me within their familiar cloak. Somewhere, (off in the distance) I heard the cows lowing.

This evening's softly lit field conveyed a distinctly different flavor from that day's brilliantly illuminated sun dance. Here now, once again, I more or less glide along in my mother-taught native Indian walk. I sense my way along (in relative blindness)—first gaining my bearings in the field that directly encompasses me, and then feeling the touch of breathing rhythms as they perpetually fill and empty around me. Location in these moments is felt more than seen; felt like Doppler echoes bouncing off walls of the waves of caves that shift in greater and lesser concentric circles that grow (surrounding me) around me.

Once again that early lesson recalled of toe first-heel gliding, in due course, led me more or less to that very place I was to be. But not, of course, without stepping into a few gopher holes, brown cow dung droppings, and vacant yellow jacket nests before I realized the fact.

Unfurl

(To be able) to travel into that scene again, where the light is so brilliant,
    it blinds momentarily
        then instantly shifts to (a disappearing pinpoint of) transfer
                . . . .whoosh!....
To trek to those places where (what considering) reality lives
    —light (years) squared—
      where one
        lives beyond the massive pull of daily gravity.
(By our sacred seas)
    To see 'n see (c times c)
      and sense once again,
        the primordial Energy of the stars that continually (light)
          phase (reflectively),
            pulse (relatively)
              in tandem,
              creating
              (super
              nova) life
              events.

          As above
          so below.

Harmonic Note

I spread my blue jacket over a little mound of earth close to the center of the field and lie back on a plot relatively devoid of gopher holes, cow dung, and yellow jackets. Evening reveries gather around me with mermaid songs, wisteria fragrances, swirling colors, and begin to compete for my attention. I search the night sky and switch back once again.

Medicine Wheel - August 1987

A couple of close friends had invited me to join them and a couple of their friends on a weekend retreat near Crabtree Falls. Janis and Erin wanted to gather a small group of us girls to help energize and celebrate a major cosmic event—the event that some said had been foretold by the ancient Maya and in the patterns of evolving stars. The Harmonic Convergence was certainly getting a lot of media hoopla of late. Supposedly, the Harmonic Convergence was to be *the* time when everyone and everything in the cosmos aligned, connected, converged over two special days in mid-August.

The media promoters of the event had even suggested that during those days the "vibes" would be just so, so that all beings and all things would be miraculously transformed (or transported) to new dimensions. The ancient Mayan prophets had predicted as much, millennia ago. Something momentous was supposed to happen to people of Earth. It was to be a worldwide happening and was firmly based on gathering top secret intelligence transmitted by our visiting, but invisible, "Space

Brothers" to those adepts who could translate the intricacies, the import, of this Knowledge.

Something like that.

I wasn't sure about what these neo-hippy, new-agey, aging hippies knew and were spreading around the globe to promote a carnival atmosphere of group meditations. But on the other hand, I knew I could sure use a nice weekend vacation in those Blue Hills once again!

I was not at all unfamiliar with the area that Janis and Erin had selected for our weekend retreat. My computer sales territory had had me crossing the Blue Ridge backbone many times over the past few years. Before that, through the 1970s between times of undergraduate and graduate schoolings, I had set up a few homes, each one on one or the other side of the ridge. Before that, in the late 1960s and early 70s, I had traveled across the Appalachians to meet my husband-to-be at university dances and where we had started our youthful, hopeful beginnings. That promising effort, in its turn, would later result in one failed married life, but resolved amicable divorce.

By the time Janis and Erin invited me to participate in their weekend gathering of friends, I was already well past the grieving of the failure of my second marriage and going nuts sublimating my energies into national account telecommunications sales. For a 30-something woman in the 1980s, the siren call of business bleated loud and clear. And like any other red-blooded American of the time, woman or man, I grabbed for the golden-tinted brass ring. Stockbrokers, limited partnerships, realtors, suitors and lovers all loved me in those days because I was making powerful money over those years.

At eighteen, suddenly left alone to forge my own way in the world, I had to learn early how to survive. Survival, the school of hard knocks taught me, pivoted around the holy trinity of an advanced education, a bottomless checkbook, and wearing a pleasing personality and appearance.

Oh, and there was a fourth commandment as well—remembered deeply from my childhood days—thou shalt maintain thy silence under any and all conditions that even remotely connect you to the non-rational worlds of the silly psychic stuff.

By the time I arrived to our campsite late that first afternoon, I had met, excelled, and vowed to maintain all four strategic-for-survival-of-life criteria. They had served me and preserved me over the years. Why rock the boat now? But I had to admit to myself, silently again, that I would observe the weekend goings-on with interest. After all I still was, as always, hugely curious.

I was eager to join my friends for a weekend in the country. Three of us had rented cabins at the Crabtree Falls campground and two other girls had decided to set up camp with tent and sleeping bags. I had left my two cats with a sitter and been purposely, deliciously ambiguous as to when I would be returning home. Janis had given me directions to the campground. It was a somewhat familiar yet altogether a new route, taking me up from the valley entrance rather than down from the mountain ridge that I was more experienced with. I had taken most of that particular road twice over two years previously, driving from Richmond to enjoy week-long intensive retreats with good folks and good minds in the mountains near Charlottesville. Janis's directions were similar to that route, except the turn from the main road was a slightly different switch that had me meandering for the first time across the Tye Valley countryside.

So on that peak of summer day in 1987, I learned yet another route to the Falls. This would be the same route I would take eleven years later when the call came through for me to return. But at that time, I didn't connect the road with its proximity to other roads, other journeys taken, nor with ones I would take later in my life. Instead, the road lulled me with its gentle sloping hills and rich panoramic vistas, and I was just grateful to leave the cares of the hectic workweek behind for spell.

The reigning valley homesteads dotted the countryside every mile or so, as the road followed the river in its course and was often crisscrossed by its flow. In preparation for the harsh winter months ahead, those homesteads with cattle farms had already harvested bales of hay into neat square bundles that clustered along fence lines or sat at regular spaces in the fields, waiting to be congregated. The farther west I drove, the more striking the contrasts between valley and hills and the wealth or lack of it that portrayed the American Dream in the mid-1980s. After ten miles or so as the crow flies, the rich, golden flatlands gave way to luxuriant, wooded, tangled undergrowth that had marked perennial Appalachian poverty for centuries. It was a surreal study of vivid contrasts, one that would haunt me for many years to come. In retrospect, it symbolized the beginning of my climb up the hills once again to the source I had all but forgotten, and to where my family and friends and roots and branches were already gathering.

Blue Hills Diary

PART II: SPIRALS OF WHEELS AND RINGS

Traveling

I travel through towns and cities recognized only by human mass magnitudes of buzzing emotions and fruitless activities and find relief in the still sacred resting points of in-between. I am named Wanderer—a traveler set into perpetual motion like a spinning top. No roots of my own are planted deeply into any single earthly human place, for these ceaseless journeys remind me to find placement in the branches of the unseen, where the whirlwind dances surround any one now, and any now called Home.

Home is sanctuary—it is the place where life travels take an exit off of the common ramp; the place for when we choose to take rest for a spell. If lucky, I could call a dwelling place "my home" for more than a couple of years. By my 35th year, when I traveled to the Harmonic Convergence (returning once again) to sanctuary called the Blue Hills, I could already claim eighteen homes once rented or owned. After a remarkably rootless childhood of being transplanted now and again (to follow yet another promising garden called paradise) and feeling more and more as though in perpetual motion due to one family crisis or another (events beyond my child control), the theme of traveling had been well ingrained. These—my childhood family homes—would distance four points of the compass across America and reach more or less haphazardly into anonymous metropolises, gossipy burghs, and the wide expanses of reclusive no-where lands. While longitude and latitude crosshatches could map this journey according to raw physical geography, nothing could compare to the climatic emotional undercurrents that would come to be associated (memories) with each of these temporary plantings.

Today when I recall my early half-life years, what billows forth to fill my memory are those prevailing whirlwinds of yesterdays. Each center of recall brings back currents of times spent in dwellings well remembered, not for their sanctuary, but for their perpetual shifts of emotional climate and the question of whether or not I could survive. For Dad (and in the beginning, Mom), each new home offered the promise of a new dawn, surrounded by an aura of anticipation toward future possibilities and potentials yet to become.

> But each golden promise
> (dreamy tales in perpetual circles of mistaken appointments)
> would return to lead again
> (repetitive grooves of well worn life records)
> to yet another tale of tally ho! forged akashic annals of gambles taken
> (those seemingly all or none choices by chance)
> which in turn become first divided, then lost, forgotten thence scattered
> (ashes of hope and musing reminders of our celestial dance)
> color rhythm movement added to drab sepia-toned faded bygones
> already rented and mortgaged *words* now nowhere conceivable or viable options remain to
> repair the
> seams for rejoining.

An Aside

Each new home, each relocation, fostered such excitement and anticipation for us. It was as if we were witnessing once again (at aurora's first blushing promise of a new dawn) a new page turning of another chapter in the book of life. Eventually, however, we came to the realization that each movement, each home sanctuary in life travels (encompasses) its own design upon our psyches. That is, each promise proffers its own source of mood, color, tone, notes, songs and a series of dancing rhythms (motifs from which to connect outside) of our day to day.

Duties call (a series of never-ending lifeboat drills in retrospect) spoken silent within the struggles of a young girl's fractured remembrances, now revisited in full bloom of (a somewhat) carefully aged mid-(life)

Crisis?

Well, okay, if you must put a label on my meandering the quintessential labyrinth experience simply called "Life." One word is as good as another to classify this book of me. And perhaps a similar book of you? Ah now, that would be a welcome switch backtrack, to retrospectively learn from another's lessons offering 20-20 hindsight of reflective moonday morning quarterbacking. Whatever those concepts mean to you. It does salve and save our precious hides at times to just have a good talk or write journal notes to oneself, check the dream worlds, and catch the themes and reruns that continue to grab one out of the everyday sombulance called sleep.

Our simple notes where we refuse to be labeled for expediency and offers of pigeonholes to serve our increasing discomfort?   Well, sir and ma'am, such is our take on a life (it seems) as we turn leaves of pages of our lives.

> Go figure!

Where the new year of millennial promises of resurrected hope, 2000, rolls across the board, and those years even more so we still rile when classified into a tidy little manageable category bounded with fancy boarders as bonded to Saturn's borders?

The Sabbath on, oh, rings of Saturday or source of galactic centered Sunday?

> Go figure.

The codings are as personal as Aquarian Ganymede's cup to the gods and as playful as Falstaff's commentary in Shakespeare's second of the seventh day of rest. Perhaps the days these days of the new year (with an unexpected leap day)

> we'll signal our renewal for a 2001 space odyssey?

Well dears, again, I seem to have gotten off track in my topic of traveling and perpetual motion and so will backtrack, return to the place where I last left off, and where delays and explanations are infinitely necessary to weave this story of the Blue Hills. That title concept is as good as another and builds on the foundation of singular memories in retrospect, summed from the events and experiences now in hindsight, called wisdom of maturity.

    At 46 today, these recollections of those earlier days rush forth well-bidden with all of the vivid intensity of virtual reality known as then and there.

    What we call roots and home—a relative relationship—
>first becomes fractures for healing,
>>remembered in retrospective
>
>motion musings
>(backward forwards inside out).
>>Born to a life of (sensed
>>perpetual) rootlessness,
>
>sentient travelers paradoxically move inside most moments
>>>(a snapshot still to life)
>>>of Now.

    With growing familiarity, we catch glimmers first, and then begin to recognize our secret passage between here and there, one that calls and conveys us to our travels yet once again.

Medicine Wheel 1987

I began to climb out of the rich valley and onto that twisty mountain road (that led up) to the Appalachian campground. About halfway up to the summit of Crabtree Falls (where I had once hiked the Meadows along the upper crest of the Blue Ridge Parkway), the road uphill once again paralleled in my slow climb to meet the more rapid downstream (twisty returns) of the Tye River. For the first time, I missed the sudden < left into the campground area on the first pass, and needed to circle back to locate the entrance again. But once I located the entrance, it was a straight shot to the large pine log building marked OFFICE where I was to (check in and) pick up my cabin keys.

No keys were needed.
My papers and billings were already in order.

Sticky from the humid drive, I asked immediately for directions to the bathhouse where I could freshen up before the evening gathering at the campground. The owners were very accommodating, pointing out the lay of the land, the bathhouse and the general direction of my weekend cabin, including parking space. I was delighted to learn that our cabins were along the riverbank, and that we were just an easy stone's throw from the upper mountain road and the lower river depths.

It promised to be a marvelous (peak) summer

weekend of recreation, relaxation and reflection. We were each (in high spirits) anticipating the weekend in front of us. Already after five o'clock, I stopped by my cabin just long enough to drop off the cooler and a canvas bag packed with a variety of shorts, jeans and T-shirts. Then, grabbing shampoo and soap, washcloth and towel, I trudged my way up to the communal bathhouse, eager to slough off layers of sweat and road dust that had accumulated on my hair and skin over the afternoon's drive from Richmond.

That was Saturday evening, August 15th. The stock market had just climbed the day before to all-time highs with explosive volumes of activity. Meanwhile, thousands of people around the world were taking time out to assemble that weekend and reflect upon the future world. Within eight to nine weeks, the stock market would take a huge crashing fall, reminiscent of Black Friday, October 1929. Within a few days, most people assembled around the world at that gossamer moment of spiritual gatherings would soon be, like me, back in the muddy pitch of day-to-day operations that, throughout history, had veiled our very souls from ourselves and devoured lives.

Nonetheless, I felt magic in the air... A stirring anticipation breezed through, reminding me to be watchful, to let down my shields and guard for a spell. It was time to play again - to run along on a different, non-scheduled track. For just this weekend, the responsible child, *cum* responsible adult, could play again in the realm of the magical child, where the silly stuff almost forgotten from a childhood lost was being invited to play once more. I granted (g-ave Maria) a song and myself (an avenue of) permission.

Ancient Melody

When I was down and out and seeking a simple refreshment of life
—a shower to be exact with the water rolling and drumming off my back—
and hair and face and
oh, my, everywhere I could get clean enough
(I would never be clean enough!)
How many times can I wash my hands?
Of the guilt? That is not a true emotion they say.
Well, give me one that is and I will symptom substitute, nonetheless I still wash my hands of the whole deal…. I did not cause IT….(or did I?)

When I was down and out and seeking a simple refreshment of life
—a shower to be exact—I entered the shower stall with my husband and scrubbed, scrubbed with a loofah, (hoohah!) those parts of his and parts of mine that made use squeaky clean and playful then….
Back track, rewind, flooding memories look out!
The feet, my feet, the loofah fell to the floor and, my being blind, felt my way in the dark.
We were granted (by special admission) a ticket to the chamber to die together. The soap, human fat rendered with a sprinkle of perfume; the gentle wash cloth, a piece of remaining clothing, all we had to hold our dignity (together) at some time
(the annihilation of a people, the inquisition of others somehow different as decided by those different –

                                    so-called so, if
they called us on IT).
    I picked up the wire brush, imagining it a gentle cloth and scrubbed and scrubbed, kneeling on the floor and scrubbed his feet too
              with all the love that I could muster. We would be going out together again this time.

Medicine Wheel 1987

    Returning from the bathhouse with just my reading glasses on

              (the contact lenses needed a full sink and mirror to apply properly),

I was a bit shy of total nearsightedness, but my friends took no notice. The evening's celebrations were about to begin…

              (there was an aura of fun and playfulness all around).

Still, coming down from my drive and beginning to pick up the gentler vibes around me, I took my own sweet time meandering to change for supper

              (on a slightly different path more directly to my cabin).

About half-way over a rolling green hillock, something glimmering blue on the ground caught my eye. Continuing to towel my hair dry, I bent down to inspect (glittering, brilliant) what was reflecting the last rays of the waning sun.

A perfectly gorgeous blue feather!

It was focused directly on my path, at that moment when the evening shadows of sun and my life path were just so aligned. A shimmering blue feather with a white tip, left behind by some blue jay bird.

(Its perfect beauty captivated me.)

I picked the feather up, twirling it between my fingers and thumb, and giggled self-consciously. Such silliness for such a simple "sign" to mark my time over the weekend. By the time I had changed into fresh jeans and T-shirt, the feather had become part of my costume, placed neatly behind my right ear as some sort of funky get-up reminder of the 1960s

(that peace missed earlier in my teens for reasons of family traveling).

An Aside

In ways I can't explain, that blue feather caught my eye and my spirit. I felt I had been given a great gift when I found it glittering there just for me to find on the ground. Silly me! But nonetheless it felt special. That first evening, I placed it on my bedside table, carefully anchoring the quill under the clock. I could hear the other girls already gathering at the picnic table nearby and rushed out to join them. The sun was already setting, low across and upstream the river, and just the faintest flickers of light peeped through the trees. It had been a long day for all of us.

The swarms of mosquitoes and no-see-ems were thick and feasting on the five of us as we too sat down to enjoy our communal feast of your basic country picnic food: fried chicken, a variety of salads, homemade cookies, sodas, and lots of fresh water. Fully satisfied, we just listened (for a spell) as night gathered and the gurgles of our own contented stomachs echoed along with the ruminations of the Tye River babbling just a few feet away. The air smelled rich and ripe with neighboring wood smoke, sage, and pine tags deeply mulched into the dark soil; the sweet fragrance of wild rhododendrons and wisteria wafted higher, swimming on river updrafts born of those gentle night breezes. The flying critters (obviously already having had their fill) finally retired for the night. But, for us, after feasting and clean up, we decided to start our own roaring campfire. At last, I hoped to learn just what this whole Harmonic Convergence thing was about.

Artist Musings

The responsible child never really grows up. It seems to me as I write these words that she always sees her imperfections glaring

(looming dark, silent running)

rather than taking delight in the off the wall humor of life

(the perennial cosmic joke, drum roll please).

Less than perfect, where are the flaws in that tapestry?
May as well add a few to keep life interesting, eh?
Pick a couple of doozies to keep busy while
the gifts turn to fat and smoke and sloth and envy and much mush

(Guessing all the way for the most part.)
Easy tickets out of this life?
Well, I had excellent parental teachers.
Ah yes, I can say that it all started with those sparkling effervescent bubbles
of simple words
that stay with a child,
they wound, grant entrance, and never really leave
(words sticks like champagne to our head— those perpetual visitors).

           Mom had her baggage and Dad
had his.

    The child inherits the windy spirit of theirs and
adds a few more idiosyncrasies and so on and on and
do-loop back to reiterate and add one
    when go team is green and Spring sprints
another nine yards for a touchdown.

Life
        Millennial promises of renewed hope
            become tumultuous, struggles felt
                (only by a young girl's)
                    growing up
                (to hold fast)
                with sensitivities and blossoming
            tender years of tears
                (too much)
                    for my overly sensitive
ears to hear.

An Aside

From earliest childhood, my eyes grew less sensitive. I had difficulty focusing and the edges became fuzzy. To compensate, my ears became hyper-alert to any changes in the program of organized sound of music, allowing for the occasional odd note off key of warning. The optometrists would say that I learned to accommodate for one supposed lack by bolstering another complementary sense. By then my senses were already mixed up.

The wires were crossed.

What would they say to this? One of my high school jokes was making screeching bat cries.

Radar echoes in the dark, their pulsing fields
    are like concentric circles surrounding
personal harpo strings
    (in silence to make space and
    sense relative distances).
But that was then and now is now
    (whenever we choose n*ow to
be)*.
And these words and my song to you
    are painted color, music,
    and dancing notes;
    journal entries
    to hear, to
see, to feel in resonance.

Medicine Wheel 1987

We gathered around, all good friends, and just had a marvelous time chatting and catching up on each other's lives. Janis didn't go into a lot of philosophic, metaphysical mumbo jumbo, but did share her interpretation of what the Harmonic Convergence was all about and why it was important to participate.

In essence, we would be joining others this weekend at strategic spots around the globe to celebrate as one voice—one shared ritual to harmonize ourselves with Mother Earth. In turn, our collective harmony would supposedly have us all aligned and in harmony with the sun straight out and through the galactic center of the universe.

A pretty tall order, I thought, and what was this stuff about Mother Earth (a.k.a. Gaia) being a living being? Pretty farfetched, if you asked me. But, as Janis reminded us, the native peoples of the world had always believed that. They and their ancestors had always held a most profound reverence for Nature in all of her forms.

That particular weekend had been predicated centuries ago
    (already set in motion,
        use your own intuition, this was 1987
    after all).

It was foretold in various consciousness codes of the sun, moon, and stars – the planets too—that we

could tap into one universal song via our very own
consciousness sing along. Indeed, Mother Earth was
like (hey man, can you dig it?) our space vehicle and
we were preparing for our collective journey into the
New Age.

> The timing had to be just so,
>   and the song, right on key,
>   but together around the world we
>   would meditate
>   and converge with Earth,
>   our wave for all humanity.
> We could imagine and create the world one of
> peace and harmony
>   (songs of the 60s I did not hear)
>   and a form of space vehicle.
>   Huh? What was that you
>   say?
> Why did this feel all funny to me and yet...
>   And yet...? It felt familiar too.
>
>   I played along.

By the mid-1980s, I had independently studied
the more esoteric sciences and cosmology, as well as
case studies of parapsychology. Too, I had visited
other gathered retreats twice already (going on three
times) and met others more curious of the world
beyond the obvious mainstream version of reality.
Janis had been channeling a friendly being she simply
called "ET" for a few of us, and other channelers had
made me curious since I'd read Shirley Maclaine's
book *Out on a Limb*. I had so many questions to ask

about the paranormal—always curious!

> But never knew where to begin, because some
of my own psychic stuff
> > and mystical adventures scared me
> (silly)
> > > and others (away)… what
> > could I say?

It was like when we ask the teacher how to spell a word and she says,
> "Look it up in the dictionary!"
> > > I mean, yeah,
> > right….
> > IF I knew how to spell IT ,
> > > > then, I
> > wouldn't have to ask!
> > > You get the picture.

> Erin brought out her double terminated crystals—the ones she used in her healing therapy work—so that we could see what they looked like and "feel" their energy. The centerpiece crystal for the medicine wheel that would be the keystone for the wheel would be delivered sometime the next day by one of their friends, a guy simply named Bob. Erin had also just returned from her first week of classes with a man who claimed to study pieces of so-called Pleiadian spacecraft….

> > (Oh, wow, what the heck was I getting
> into here?

> I needed to back up a few spaces and try to just enjoy the fireside chat, toast another marshmallow and share some tall stories.)   The best I could offer were

the stories of the Monkey's Paw, fish fries on the Cranberry Lakes near Fidalgo, and suspected mermaids dressed in colors and singing out of range. Oh, and yeah, also some attempts of channeling a few acquaintances met along the way.

>   I played along.

An Aside

Extreme anguish is when you lose your first best friend just a few short years (of lifetimes) after finding her again. This subplot speaks both to haunts as well as to ancient remembrances. Give me a few moments to pick up the tempo, recall that resonant sharpness of those carving and blending memories cataloged under sadness and joy.

>   The first cut of many rips and shatters
>   that scatter and tear soul into tiny
>   pieces.
>   Mine eyes leak now in memory
>   for their 20-20 hindsight
>   and weep in
>   mystical wonder.
>
>   How many losses in one lifetime?

Ancient Memory

About the time I turned four years old, I recall standing between Dad and Mom at the edge of our new property in Anacortes. We stood in front of the gravel road that had just been laid down to access our housing development, and next to the big rounded boulder, just piercing above the earth. That boulder would in future years become Mom's sparkling silver-white granite rock garden.

We looked with pride at our freshly constructed, ready-to-move-in little wooden Brown house. It was really and truly ours! The excitement coming from Mom and Dad was palpable. Our dreams were high and mighty in those days. We were home-owners already, indeed.

The dream was swell and swelling as we stood gazing at our new home. I was dressed in pajamas and a light robe, Mom in her housedress, and Dad in his fishing slacks and sweatshirt. There, to my ☐left, directly across and lateral to me and my folks, stood another little towhead-blonde girl, about my age of four, with her parents. She stole a peek at me too. It was an instant of total recall and recognition—a flood of remembrance. Suddenly, without words spoken, we stole a glance between us from around the legs of our taller parental companions.

Silently, ever silently without words spoken
    the brief glance said it all...
        "My dear friend of ages, I finally
    meet you again!"
            I burst with the thought,

                              the glow, in
                              absolute joy of
                              direct recognition
                              of her "quality."
           "Yes, back (to you)," Mae replied
with a wink, her age-old child's radiance
more than her eyes I saw.
           "We are next door neighbors for
another round on this circuit. Look at us
now…. We are little people again, in
different forms this time, too."
                    "We are again," we
           thought in unison as one voice.

And as that was said, without words, the radiant light bowed and arched and intensified between us! It grew and swirled taller than our parents and wider than the stretch of the two driveways and shared grassy knoll of common grounds between us.

And, those words unspoken between us, thought beams of telepathy some would say, would lessen over time and become less and less frequent over our few years together as next "store" neighbors. We learned over time to communicate in the contemporary human way for our culture, using the English language. Her parents and my parents would become friends; our families as well as those around the small neighborhood would share celebrations with each other. It was the mid-1950s, when young parents shared hopes and dreams for their children, and the children played with no fear. It was paradise on earth, and yet, and yet, in that meeting with Mae, I first became fully aware of recollections of another time and place. That place and time, for which my child's mind could only conjure the words, I simply called, "Home."

Ancient Melodies

I have looked into the mirror and seen my many faces.

Haunting Melody

One of my striking vivid memories of Anacortes (Fidalgo Island USA – homesteading still allowed nearby) was the time when astronaut John Glenn orbited the earth. Three cycles, February 19th I recall. But the morning that he was to take off and launch up, up and away, I was down and out with a new "flu bug" and Glenn's travels in space were not the highlight of *my* mind in those days, to be perfectly honest. I felt absolutely miserable and took to bed early on *that particular* morning!

>The virus *they said*,
>>flush me, *they said*
>>>with lots of liquids; some asp-burns in a dot kissed with sweet watered-down sugar served on a t-spoon.

In those years - 1962 to be exact - at our house, home remedies were the cure. Don't even think that there was such a thing as Medical Insurance. Anyway, Mom and Dad had precious medical background and rather than going to the hospital, I was treated at home. Round the clock bedside care, particularly when my fever began to spike into the danger zone

—of sheesh! —
I recall 104 degrees with alcohol sponge baths and cool wet soaks.

John Glenn must have returned to Earth victorious, but by that time I didn't know and couldn't care. I was fighting for my life, and not the first time, come to think of it. One of our best family friends was the gentle neighborhood doctor. I recall him well. Dr. Noble made house-calls in those days. Maybe we ranked as a family somehow, but I was always happy to see him, through bleary eyes filled with heated fever, and sense his deepening concern for my well being.

Anyway, after a number of weeks of being bedridden with no particular certainty of diagnosis, I was allowed to move around, regain my bearings and be "normal again." Doctor Noble and my folks later gave me the diagnosis of non-paralytic polio. That diagnosis switched from flu virus, sometime during the astronaut's hurrahs and the overhead sonic booms that bounced off the walls at night in our small three bedroom home.

Dad got extra help from his ham radio (shortwave) buddies, too. K7MVZ handle with care and concern for his little girl and information located in Morse CQ to points far distant from our island neighborhood locale. His hobby, to communicate via airwaves, supported our little town hospital and Dr. Noble, whose office was next to the community park with an outdoor amphitheater, and across the street from the unusually large three-story Carnegie library. Anyhow, I healed and never forgot those tenuous times. The most wonderful part of those days, if there was one, was the special loving and caring—and discovering Nancy Drew mystery books. I read as many of those as I could to keep focus. By the time we moved to Friday Creek, I was well-versed in the keen seek-you-shall-find mysteries of the old clock and the tolling bell.

Haunting Melody

One day, seemingly out of the blue, my folks united unilaterally and decided that there was no more to be gained in the little, quiet, isolated island town named for Anna Curtis. With only a boat and a drawbridge to connect to the mainland, and a ferry boat transport to other San Juan Islands and British Columbia, life for them felt limited. So, we gathered our stuff and moved to our little bungalow home. It, too, was isolated and located somewhere between the towns of Burlington and Bellingham off Highway 99, the main road to Canada. The cottage was a rental home that once had been some sort of boarding house café. One of the most curious discoveries in this home (and it was a sanctuary for the most part to me) was a full-sized, well-polished, heavy oak bar, complete with five barstools anchored to the floor that divided the bright cheery kitchen from the more subdued communal dining area.

This move to the country would mark the first severing of a dear friendship. With barely time to say good-bye to my best friend Mae, we were whisked away to our new home.

Oh, what anguish! I was inconsolable for days
—until I met my new best friend, Lee the
tomboy and her brothers.
      Also, to make this big move even more
  tragic
     (from my point of view then and in
compassionate recall now)
          was the loss of my first kitty cat,
  Amos,

             sometime
          between then and when
         we moved..

My isolation was feeling complete. However, my parents were way too thrilled about the new home on Friday Creek, with huge wild blackberry bushes in the backyard, the pink salmon and rainbow trout runs, periwinkles, fresh mint, wild pink rosebushes, and sweet spring water to faucet directly from our own well, to pay me any mind.

    Well,

I consoled from my tears by climbing up into a simple tree house built from wooden planks with a bird's eye view overlooking Friday Creek. I would stare out from my vantage point in the tree house and watch the creek, as it first divided around a magnificent island of gravel, stone, brush and tender saplings, and then reconnected again like a two-laned highway.

    The island, formed in between
        those laughing waters that rushed
  downstream

                              over stepping stones posed by
                granite rocks,
                                    those seeming
                         barricades of life.
          And all the time, while I observed the splendor
that day
                         I salved my pain and munched my way
                              through a bag full of Brach's real
                licor ice candies.
 'Tis strange, no downright odd, the memories we
recall on moving days.

An Aside

          Oh, migod! When the reveries start to come,
they flash in floods at times. Time to take another
break for a spell. Get outside and hear the peace,
watch the birds scurry and flit to their new homes,
smell the Spring once again popping out all over

                         … It is in the very air I breathe…

Unfurl

Early life in Washington State… both places
Fidalgo Island in the archipelago of the Strait of Juan de Fuca
and
Friday Creek where there is still a mystery left < behind
over numerous scribbles and musical codes
scattered along logging and mining
old rural route Highway 99.
As are many teeny tiny splinters of memories
—backtracks of distant houses and subplots—

almost
heaven
when compared to the later moves south (CA) where it began
> then central US (ARK) for four days
> then mid-Atlantic southeast (NC) to stay put for a spell
> then north to (VA) where the agony was in earnest.
The erasure of childhood dreams upon early maturity at eighteen
plus or minus a few months.
That magic number eighteen, when new dreams are substituted
and I began my venture into early adulthood

somewhere in there.

Haunting Memory

There was a new urgency at home that Spring of 1961 when Dad and I returned from our "'cross country" drive through many of the United States to Arkansas, picked up Route 66 on return to Disneyland, California and then back up the coast to Fidalgo. (My sister and I, in retrospect, suspect that Mom was pregnant again—an unpotentiated gleam of anticipation in their eyes again—and one more baby who would never be make it to earth.) Anyway, during this fragment of time between familial hope and hopeless, the meeting of my dad with his dad in Arkansas had not been a total failure.

They finally met face to face for the first time since my birth. Yet I could feel that there was a lot of tension between them. And, when my new step-grandmother's job was to insist that my new shoes matched my fashionable ensemble, as was befitting a young Southern lady of the day, she must have thought that I was a wild thing, for I always seemed to sorely disappoint her! But for me the whole trip with my dad was a magical mystery tour comparable to the lands of Disney. What fun we had! When we returned, I was eager to show my first ever, new suntan to my friends back home, the collected "soupiners," photograph slides, and the bunches of café luncheon and dinner placemats gathered stop by stop from the various roadside eateries we visited along our journey.

Dad shared his Kodak moments with the guys at the local Elks, too.

Mom remained rather quiet those days, just

happy to have us home again where things could get back to "normal" (whatever that was).

My sister was again largely invisible, playing by herself, or with Mom, trying not to get in our way.

After a rest from the whirlwind vacation, I savored the good memories of that late summer: playing doctor, dress up, and curiously focusing on the death of a friend's pet (a solemn ceremony we neighborhood children held in remarkable reverence and weeping for Sox's good, short, doggie life).

Then, without warning, it was suddenly time to move to the little bungalow home before the Fall, before beginning again, another transition to another school year.

And then the fifth grade began. It was an exhaustingly long bus trip to and from the country school, particularly when I was lugging Mom's violin (most precious, she named it Andre) back and forth from stop to stop, as well as a bag full of books. That school year, too, was shortened in late Winter, when my dad, who was always trying to improve our condition, found out that he was not suited for Private Eye or Insurance work. He had encountered a string of failed jobs. Not many jobs in the rustic country, he said. So we had to move on again, and quickly.

Money was running out!

We had to auction off everything we owned just to live, pick-up and go.

Everything!

The most traumatic thing of all was the auction of all we had, including Mom's copper plates of the famous composers that she had on the wall... that made her cry most of all, I recall. Our precious stuff "all-gone" for each of us, except for clothes we wore and two grocery bags each to stuff into the car, our Rambler American

> (its color called "desert sand"—a presentiment of moves to come).

The German Shepherd, sweet Andy, and her remaining fat pup,

> Blue, to stay with Lee's family -
> (their Springer Spaniel having rights of paternity, the father of Blue).

I still mourned the loss of our black and white kitty cat, Amos. A hurt deep inside that held no answers. She supposedly got lost somewhere in between our move from Fidalgo to Friday Creek—she never made that incredible journey.

And Henry James Sylvester Bird-Brain Brown, our blue and yellow parakeet, bit the dust just a few weeks earlier. I discovered him DEAD one day at the bottom of his cage; his timing seemed to be a portent (in retrospect) of our family transition from joy to sorrow. His silent song would speak more than any words we could say to each other in the agonizing slow death of our family over the days to come.

My mother was beside herself with the sudden shift. We had to move again, away from our bungalow home nestled serenely in its wooded paradise. Dad had to run the auction of what was left of our belongings and furniture. I got to keep my scrapbook and international stamp album. In "trade" and in gratitude to our home, I hid clues of my life – bits of stories and musical notes written wedged behind the wallpaper and in basement hidey-holes. I wonder today if they are still there. My sister retained her little black dog toy, Douglas, I recall. Actually, Douglas was a favorite childhood stuffed toy for both of us, and her choice made me glad. Throughout it all, Dad tried to keep a stiff upper lip, but no lie, it was hell for all of us.

Why in the world would we have to leave that wonderful heaven on earth? Why move again? And why be wrenched away from another best friend and far, farther away from Mae and Anacortes friends? California sounded like fun (and it was advertised as such and I had been there once) but, but, arghhh, it just did not make sense. But we all loved that home at Friday Creek.

I still wonder about the "why" of it. Why move at all? And why all so sudden and urgent? I did not understand. I would find out over the years that every move, every transition in my life would take on this same dramatic pace of "about face." In reflection, there has been nothing smooth and gradual concerning change in my life.

We had become attached to our home near Friday Creek. We had endured the Great October Columbus Day storm of 1962 and survived that hurricane night. Dad was almost electrocuted when the electricity grounded through the kitchen sink drain. Mom covered the windows with blankets to prevent potential shattered glass from flying into the rooms of the cottage. The creek overran its banks the next day, swelling deep into the backyard, threatening our open basement. And the power lines crashed onto the firs and pines across Highway 99, igniting a forest fire among those very trees where Mom and I had taken so many of our Indian walks. Dad had to drive through the height of the storm into town to notify the volunteer fire fighters. The phones lines, too, were down.

During the height of the wind and before the forest fire and drenching rain, I wanted to be outside to feel the wind on my face. I made a run for it! And quickly discovered that the wind was more powerful than this ten-year-old girl. Luckily, before I literally flew off to God knows where, Dad rescued me and carried me back into the house to safety.

These types of events can flood every person's life recall when we reminisce on our early days. But beyond the events, there are the feelings attached—

feelings of danger, sorrow, anticipation, and sometimes, exquisite joy.
Like when Mom sung on her violin.

And the great sadness I felt to leave Lee and her brothers behind. I never saw them again. I never saw Mae again either, although we did get a chance to play in the tree house, swim and raft the creek, and fill big coffee cans full of blackberries that first and only summer.

Dad dropped us off in Waverly, Oregon, at Mom's parents' home, and then continued south to California. Mom's parents were caretakers of the land. Grandpa's green thumb and gentle words encouraged the most magnificent rose, shrub, and vegetable gardens; the land spanned acres. He sculpted the holly bushes and hedgerows along their own design, allowing them to follow the lines of the land. By the time we arrived, the vineyards were already mature, tamed to their poles and overflowing with grapes of many varieties and flavors. I would follow him everywhere, as did his menagerie of dogs, while he made his daily rounds. Gramsie would visit the children, taking time to read to them, then taking us all out for a picnic or a swim in one of the huge in-ground swimming pools.

As caretakers, Gramsie and Grandpa were given a large home of their own to maintain and enjoy. For those weeks in transition, Mom, Kathryn and I stayed in a little apartment, a flight above the "safari" ballroom filled with stuffed exotic animal heads, where I would roller-skate around "the rink" and pat each one on the nose in turn. This ballroom *qua* skating rink, in turn, had been built over the horse stables that no longer held horses, but instead, housed Grandpa's flock of goats. It was a fairytale place for me to be, while Mom missed Dad terribly and became morose, and toddler sister slept and wailed, alternately tired and cranky. In the evenings, I buried my nose in books to escape. I had discovered the new Trixie Beldon mysteries...no Nancy Drew books around in the little library downstairs adjacent to the ballroom.

(I did discover one Hardy Boys mystery book, and
> a really haunting scared-to-my-wits book about Pan—that goat-
>> man creature—you know, the one with the hoofed-feet.)

This then, my spring of discovery,
> and there when Dad was hunting for a job in sunny Californ-I-A , searching for the golden-ring in the big city of L.A.

I realize today that Dad was always looking for a "better" job. He said his greatest liability was no college degree, and yet he was so talented and versatile. He was always looking for something more. Could it be, I wonder— was he searching for that intangible, mystical, "More?" Because of his search for some personal grail, we moved often and like nomads, with little more than the clothes on our back, throughout my childhood days.

> I got used to it.
>> I played along.

Harmonic Note

My Mother and sister played virtuoso violin, while I played second fiddle in the symphonies of life, until I realized music comes in many forms of expression connected between ear and heart.

Medicine Wheel 1987

Our campfire quickly roared into life. Smoking, crackling and flaming as tiny sparks flew out and sputtered around our heated, unearthly, glowing faces. The night was already sleeping, a deep shadowy black had descended all around us as we five sat surrounding that lively, sweet oak and maple fire. We took turns and told our stories late into the night, sharing updates of lives characteristic for women in their mid-thirties. But a lot discussed was quite uncharacteristic too, obviously, with a chief accountant (an ET channeler), a new mother (a healer), two talented artists moving to Santa Fe, and me. What a mix! It was a wonderful, most memorable night of gab, and just having that special sense of freedom that only the depths of night and a roaring campfire conducive to imagination and vivid storytelling can give.

I lit my second cigarette for the evening and watched its blue smoke swirl, dance, and then join and blend with the more fragrant smoke being continuously released by the larger campfire. I told the girls about my encounter with the blue feather earlier that evening. Surprisingly, nobody laughed. Instead, I was encouraged to wear that feather the next day as a kind of signal to the powers that be that I was fully with the program.

That evening, sitting around our sparking campfire surrounded by ripe rhododendrons and sweet piney spruce, we listened to the chatter of the enveloping protective night and kicked back, fully caught in the moment. Our laughter rang through the valley hills in anticipation of the next day's ceremony of the Medicine Wheel. No doubt about it, we five were already bonding a group identity. We had come together through something powerful, meaningful and purposeful to meet at that time and place. I felt that we had already begun our own passage into Harmonic Convergence!

As our campfire slowly glowed down to the embers, we all hugged and said our goodnights. Wonderfully exhausted from the laughter, the food and the fragrant, clear night air, I slept like a baby that night. Something really magical was in the air and I couldn't wait to see what the next day would bring. Returning to my cabin, I took the blue feather from behind my ear and secured it under the clock by my bedside. With a smile of gratitude to the powers that be for this excursion weekend, I immediately fell into a deep, dreamless sleep.

Ancient Melodies

> I travel many times of now
>   simultaneously, in tandem,
>   to re-call that,
>   what? already enfolded
>   —planted   eons
>   ago—
>   deep
>   within my stillness
>   center.
> Silent core unfolds petal enfolds,
>   and re-members those
>   elemental roots
>   branching
>   backward, forward,
>   (inside out) and
>   Homeward
>   to the stars.

Medicine Wheel 1987

After a simple breakfast of bread, jam and some apple, we cleaned the table again and took turns getting dressed and playing with Erin's new baby boy. He would remain secured in his car seat on top of the picnic table on the near shore, while we would cross and re-cross the Tye River several times that Sunday, August 16th. A great baby, Erin's boy, giggling and gurgling and peeing and pooping all through the day. Each of us was drawn to the little guy, four childless women and a suddenly new mother. Each, in her own way, delighted him with chatter and attention.

And then there was Bob. A funny, rather nomadic kind of guy, he was. A friendly friend of Janis and Erin's. Bob kept the city of Richmond stocked with crystals mined from the deep caves of the ancient Ozark mountains. He had arrived sometime during the wee hours of the morning to join us, and was still sleeping on the picnic table that early morning dawn with a guitar, knapsack and a beautiful Arkansan crystal in tow. Janis had selected and purchased that magnificent, multifaceted crystal just a few days before. It was to be the centerpiece of our efforts, the hub of our medicine wheel, the *pièce de résistance* of our joint contribution to the ceremony taking place that weekend around the globe.

And, similar to a woman wearing the best of fashion designers Calvin or Ann Klein or even Yves St. Laurent, I wore my blue feather, again tucked behind my right ear, proudly that day. Me, unexpectedly remembering an ancient Indian woman back to the times when rituals really meant something. I was getting that flavor, that remembrance, because it was all around me with my friends and had spread among us like a contagion. The ritual tobacco leaves of the Virginias-Carolinas were in turn tucked under each of the carefully selected and placed stones of the wheel. The concentric rings of stones were constructed carefully to mark the directions of the four pillars, the four earthly-cosmic energy sources. We gathered the most unique rocks we could find, many resting silently yet strangely calling to us from along the far shore of the river. The center of placement for the medicine wheel we had scouted out by various means and discovered together. The "perfect place", our sacred place, was located in a tiny grassy meadow nestled deep within the dense tangle of trees and shrub, well hidden on the other side. In order to build it, we crossed and re-crossed the Tye River many times that day.

The Well

When I am lacking I go to the Source. It alone is inexhaustible, the unchangeable within the change amidst the chaos that lives in the confusion above. I drink thirstily from its fresh deep waters to find my own connection in Nature's order, and once again penetrate the universal truths that link with hearts and minds of others.

I slept wonderfully that night and woke before dawn, already anticipating the day ahead. Glad to have the soda machine nearby, I made two trips there before the rest of the world woke up. As I readied myself for the day, the early warming mists continued to rise and began to roll golden light over the distant hills. Across the highway, the valleys were still under the deep silver spell of sleep, like some Beauty awaiting her Prince's magical kiss to dispel the vapors gathered overnight. Ed (a.k.a. LateKnight) and I already missed each other. His hospitals' support work held him from taking this trip with me this time. I was alone in my travels and lovingly supported by him throughout their duration. It promised to be yet another record hot humid day on the road again in the mid-90s in the middle of September. I wondered where to drive that morning—should I go back to Dianne's cabin to reflect or go directly to the Falls? I decided to just start out and go where the mood pulled me, leaving slightly after eight a.m. I had made plans for later in the day, but this morning I had a big chunk of precious morning time all to myself. By the time I came to the decision point to turn right to Dianne's cabin or left to the Falls, there was no question. I took the road across the wide harvest valley and began the steep mountain climb of the Falls.

All the while along the drive, I asked for some time alone with my magic mountain area. I especially wanted that day to get back into that (butterfly) space—the one captured and held dearly, close to me, just the day before. Important, to receive those private moments; it was vitally important to me somehow, in some way that I couldn't yet know, to fathom its depths.

I had traveled a bit of a distance to be present at this mountain area for those two days. Every year or so for the past two decades, there were various reasons to visit. Yet over the years of 1997 and 1998, the reasons to revisit, reconnect continued to grow stronger. I felt that I was becoming already long overdue. The siren call came early that September and it could not be ignored any longer. Now, as I recall and revisit these words in December, it was most essentially a time to remember. But I am getting ahead of myself again. More than anything, I simply wanted to be alone once again to commune and find that peace of nature that those Blue Hills always seemed to grant me. A wish, a short wave of a magical hand, and I had been transported to this place once again. I did not want to feel foolish or self-conscious during those times of quiet reflection. I usually felt the need to apologize when tuning-in, turning space-y, with other folks around. My eyes would gaze at some distant sight or my ears attune to some distant music that, in reality, (which reality?) was not present in the present we shared, but nevertheless, I heard and saw.

The Butterflies

Rationally, I figured that this day being a Tuesday before the leaves changed again and before the tourist peak of the year, I had a good chance to get my wish. I was glad that I had chosen to visit in the off season—a holiday for me. For most everyone else, it would be a workday. What a gift! Such freedom! The journey was a gift to myself. Not merely a few times in that early September of 1998 did I wonder. Whatever it was, the incredible, magnetic pull I felt to visit this area at that time was captivating.

It had been gathering and building over several months and the intensity could no longer be ignored. The day before, on the path up to observe the Falls (where I had been several times before), was an adventure, and then to return to witness the birthing and blossoming of those newly metamorphosed butterflies! Well, deep inside me the meaning of the timing of the place was becoming crystal clear. Their universal symbol of change and transformation—their newfound, flying freedom and exquisite beauty; their unfettered playfulness, yet directed innate inner sense of purposefulness—was not lost on me.

As the iridescent blue butterfly transfigures— from essential ground and rock hugging (ugly to some) caterpillars into a huge shift of perspective, where beauty is free to live on both ground and in air—did she still recall (her former life)?

Did she recall the pain and the shearing off of her old bodies over all of her stages of life that were solely necessary? Only to then, at those times, be exquisitely vulnerable, as her ever-widening vision evolved to become? Was that her delight I was *seeing* as she moved in and out drawing nectar from the multitude of yellow-orange flowers?

Even more pensive thoughts continued to come to me. Were those few iridescent blues who ventured off their safe butterfly island home to meet me, inspect me the day before, somehow drawn to me as I sat seated on my stony perch on the shore desiring to draw them? Were those rare few sojourners simply the more adventuresome of the lot?

It did seem for a few moments the day before that they were most willing to call me into their world, their wide web of being. Somehow, some way, together we had created a interface between us and constructed a mutual bridge of *seeing* that brighter light. A bridge of light that allowed us to communicate freely between the gulf of creatures we think we are. It was with these curious thoughts and feelings that I turned into the vacant parking lot that morning. The Appalachian hiking trails were clearly marked with their associated campsites, but I would not be taking them that day. The sun was just moving into the early rising sky and hovering, shimmering directly along the Tye River to the left in front of me. And the warming river breezes shuffled soundlessly once again.

Haunting Melody

Between our family moves from Washington State
    to Washington District of Columbia (south
Arlington to be more exact),
        our family of four was called south to
    sunny California
                with its glitzy trumped up
          glamour
                (Hollywood stars,
                Disneyland
                fantasy lands, and
                sweet scented
                orange blossoms
                and lemon citrus
                groves, oh my).

        A child's dream!
 Yet, between the Washingtons
    certain melodies (those non-mellow dramas)
        remain ever sour and painful.
Wounds cut deeply into my psyche (the first cut is the
deepest)
    and relief is not remedied by popping a pill for
heartburn either.

Seeking Solitude

When I pulled into the Crabtree Falls parking area that Tuesday morning, I saw that there were no other cars in the lot. What absolute joy to know at that moment there would be no other people hiking, wandering, wanting to talk! I had asked for a private space of time to commune (instead) with this mountain.

Sweet silence, pure serenity, pristine clarity.

All around, as far as I could see, the gift of that early morning (unfoldment) was granted. It seemed so special in a way, to feel wholly attuned with dawning Nature as she awakened that morning. It was like getting to one's very own safe place, home base—on time, in synch—a home run. Something greater than my own scheduled planning was at work. Even then, I knew that.

Easy too, to simply to let the spirit guide me that morning, no clocks, no timetable, no particular limitations of where, when (there, then) to be. Total trust, come what may, had been the only order of the day. So here I was, having no other desire, no other particular aims or wishes except to be at that mountain once more, again.

After all, I had promised them—the mountain, the river, the waterfalls, the butterflies, bridge, paths, rocks, thickets and island—that I would return that morning.

Medicine Wheel 1987

The Tye River was low enough that late summer so that we all had a widely spaced step stone path of rocks we could take across the river to the other side. How convenient! Those rocks were slippery, and a few would stutter, unstable under our feet. We got our ankles and calves wet, too, at one time or another when we went sloshing up and down the rocks like nanny goats. We would try to grab the rocks with our toes through the soles of our sneakers and well, some of those times we just did not grab well enough and an ankle or knee would submerge into the surrounding cool eddies. That was just fine for us, for the day was sunny, sparkly and already quite hot again. An occasional dip into the river was refreshing rather than a problem.

For the others anyway.

I still had my problem with vertigo and preferred to take my time and to be sure I was on solid ground or stable rock before taking the next step. That made me painfully, painfully slow and (obvious to any watcher) careful in my river crossings. Yet, once I was securely on one shore or the other I would feel a sense of relief, sighing heavily, always preferring to spend my time (then) solidly on *terra firma*.

We spent most of the day enjoying our treks back and forth, stopping for some lunch, minding the baby, casting off a layer of clothes as the day heated up, or simply running into the deeper woods to pee. I followed with great interest the construction of our medicine wheel, the different meanings that corresponded to the placement of the stones and what, in effect, we were creating together as our legacy to the Harmonic Convergence.

The day of building had not been without mishaps, however. Besides some of the slipping and sliding off of the bridge of rocks, the girls, save me, were badly stung by yellow jackets when one foot or the other slipped not onto the pebbly soil above the water, but directly into a yellow jacket nest. An angry bee would somehow find its way up a tied down pant-leg or down under a sock and sting the beejesus out of Erin, Janis or one of their friends. We would hear a screech of surprise and pain and then all come running to help pull the still pulsing bee and stinger out of a leg, a thigh or an ankle. Nasty, tearful pain, our only remedy the cool Tye River water, a sweet mountain leaf, and a paste of mud and water.

For me, a sting could have been deadly (so my father had told me). I had grown up watching him panic like a baby whenever a bee flew unawares into our car. Also my own sting on my foot when I was around four or five had left the area puffed and me sick for days with the admonition to never get close to a bee again. Somehow in my careful (Indian) walk I had missed those nests.

                Perhaps my blue feather had protected me.
                        Who knows?
        (We hadn't even considered that they would be a problem.)

But the bees and their stings paled in contrast with the growing realization that we had done it! Together we had created and built something pretty far-out and important that day, connecting us to others around the world with a vision of peace and harmony. We each had contributed to the construction of our own little part of it and in so doing so, we had all together accomplished something that stretched timeless memories between us; collectively together we had learned something priceless.

After we re-crossed the river for the last time that day, we rested for a spell and then gathered together for our evening meal. The brilliant sunlight of that day was already diffusing through the late afternoon humid haze, giving way to the low lights of glimmer peeking between the shores, through the canopy of dense trees upstream. Janis and Erin were already rapt in discussion and seemed to be chanting together.

>They were asking the Queen of the Bees,
>>the divas (they called them)
>>>to allow us to be on their land
>>without being harmed.
>>>>We mean no harm (they chanted),
>>>>>only that we were
>>>>>sorry to be so clumsy
>>>>as to have stepped directly into
>>>your yellow jacket homes.
>
>We will be more careful the next time.
>>A truce of sorts was called that night between us—

                    we the invading humans and
        they the bees.

    From then on, although the bees would fly and scatter around that evening and the next day, not one of us would be stung again during the remainder of that weekend.

    This way of communication with bee devas and nature spirits (the wee ones) was a new one for me.

                    I played along.

    I didn't understand, but it seemed to work. No one reported any more stings over the rest of the weekend. Nor did I understand that we *could* (really?) *talk* to these nature spirits in any way, shape or form.

        A major learning experience—one lesson
            that years into the future
                I would continue to follow
                    whenever I journeyed
                    into a homeland of
                    another
                        (consciousness).
        First taught by my mother,
            a reminder from those dense
        forests walks along Friday Creek,
            the Golden Rule toward all Life,
                    in reverence,
                simply said, "Do no
                harm."

Fairy Ring 1997

Coincidentally, it was a weekend in August, exactly ten years later, when the wee ones and otherworldly concentric wheels moved back into my consciousness. I had been working nonstop on a World-Wide-Web project, rooted and planted for the past several days inside the chambers of my office, and would not have noticed anything out-of-doors, except that Ed came home from work early one morning and asked me to follow him outside. There was something he wanted me to see in our front lawn.

Ohmigod! What the world was this marvel I was seeing?! As clearly and plainly as seeing a tree or a house or a desk, I saw with my own two eyes a series of concentric circles etched deeply into the grass! Approximately two and one-half feet in perfect diameter, they rested in the center of our front lawn and yet not could be seen from the house or road. You would have to be almost on top of them to see, but the circle, there it was! No mistake, it was clear to see! Such a simple yet distinctive design! The center area for about one and one-half feet was your basic clover and crabgrass, encircled by a ring of dead grass and dirt, then a width of four to six inches of healthy green grass *flattened in the same clockwise direction* all around! Working outward to the perimeter, there was another couple of inches of dead grass and dirt that completed the outline of the circle, thus distinguishing the overall concentric rings' design from the rest of the basic clover and scrub grass of the yard.

I was speechless at the sight of it and full of questions at the same time. Ed said that he had noted it the day before while mowing the grass and had carefully bypassed the arrangement until I could get a chance to see it. Was it a fairy ring, a mini crop circle, or a tiny medicine wheel? As my scientific mind went into gear, I logically began to try reasoning the experience as soon as the initial shock of the experience wore off to some degree and I could gather my wits around me. My logic went something like this: Well, science's explanation of fairy rings in nature is that they are typically around and/or spawned by mushrooms. There were no mushrooms around to be seen before, during or after. Mushrooms rarely if ever erupted in our yard and further, we had been having a dry spell that summer.

But my heart and soul were dancing! What incredible magic had just appeared in our yard? Did it relate to the crop circles because of the flattened grass? Was it a psychic reminder of the medicine wheel of rings we girls had created ten years earlier? Was it a psychic emanation, that is, a "thought" made manifest, tangible, and if so, where or who did it come from? And why, always the why? And why then, and why the recognizable shape, and why the different textures, and why a symbol that was meaningful to both Ed and me? For him, it was a reminder of the fairy rings of old; the "little people" had left their mark and graced our land. We needed to show our appreciation with a little gift of cereal and milk that night. For me, my gut reaction was that it was the medicine wheel reminder, even though medicine wheels and those days in the Blue Hills were far from my mind during those intensive days of writing Web pages and emails and data interpretation. And in my mystical place of mystery, I could not help wondering whether it might have something to do with those tiny, glittering brighter than bright, lights that I sometimes saw domed overhead at our home against the bright blue daylight sky.

There were layers of synchronicity raveling and unraveling for me when I first saw the rings. These questions rose quickly in a jumble all into my conscious mind and I had a lot of intensity about the whole thing. Later that night, after feeding the wee ones (or the neighborhood cats!) their milk and cereal, synchronicity continued in full force, as if there was something there (a lesson?) not to be forgotten. Around midnight, I picked up my mystery book to relax and began reading again. Within a couple of paragraphs, I startled and could only say,

"Ohmigod, Wow! Ed listen to this!" I bounded out of bed and read him those couple of the paragraphs that had just smacked me broadside, over the head, and into my depths of inner resonance.

It was a story of a woman who honors her tribe's wee folks and feeds them tobacco so that they will never forget her. The story talked of human time and the timelessness of the other worlds of being, how we leave each other reminders on occasion, not to forget our relationship and vows to each other. Well, that blew my mind for both the timing of the rings that day and reading about something so similar that evening, even when in an attempt to change the subject. Evidently, the Universe was still holding on, and the so-called library angel had dropped just the appropriate book off for the realization of it all. I still do not have the answers to my many questions of how and why. But something was grabbing my attention and the tangible and intangible were working in tandem that day and night.

I felt ever so blessed, as did Ed, for he too found *his* inner meaningfulness confirmed in the ways that each of us, only from the depths of our own resonance, knew. But we knew we shared something sacred and powerful, here and together, and that design of alternating rings and wheels etched deeply into the ground stayed with us, with minimal fading, for exactly six months.

And then one day they were simply gone.

Haunting Melody

Happy life at our country bungalow home along Friday Creek, where the salmon run home to spawn and die, lasted less than a year. The auction was unbearable, traumatic; for it marked not only the loss of most everything we owned, it the beginning of our family's tumble down, a long fall from which we as a family would not return. The before and after is clear to see today in retrospect. But when we were in the midst and mist of tumbling, rolling, and roiling down that waterfall of life, there wasn't much to sight-see and life thereafter held for us few Kodak moments. By then, Mom had lost her babies not-to-be-born and the sudden uproot from our country sanctuary had pretty much done her in. From there on out, life became daily trials of survival for her; and as the joys diminished, so did she, and the unconsciousness of death began to beckon.

The South Gate of the City of Angels was a horrendous time, and beers could not quench her thirst. Dad retreated to his clay modeling statues hobby (a renaissance rebirth of sorts) and a personnel job with a company in Vernon. Mom and Dad affectionately called each other Bulldog (a name I know not the source of, except, perhaps, for their tenacious hold onto life and each other).

The South Gate apartment was tiny for us four. My sister rarely ventured outside (she was clumsy in her stride) and I roller skated circles (chased my tail and trails) around the driveway, and sometimes ventured up and down the sidewalks

>   (avoiding the cracks to spare my
> mother's back).

Then, one night when Dad was away, a priest came to our door. Mom wanted to partake of the sacrament again, but the Church had excommunicated her. (Dad's first marriage had been annulled, it didn't count in the eyes of civil law, but that made no difference to Church law, it seemed). A last straw of hope in Mom, for she was desperately begging, trying to hold on to that one soul's remaining cry for help ....

>   but in quiet tones the priest said: No can do.

She was forever to live in that no-woman's land of purgatory; unrecognized by the Church, her daughters born in sin

(or was it hell and limbo? I haven't kept up with those most recent papal decrees). What cruelty—to abandon one of the shepherd's flock! But no amount of pleading or heart cries would change the judgment.

>   It was sin and it was so.

Holy Mother of God, she was lost, lost without a straw to hang onto and spiraling down fast; totally abandoned by her God and any hope of redemption. I was about twelve then

>   (no longer afraid to roller skate over cracks to spare my mother's back,
>   as she had been crushed and chopped to bits that evening
>   thoroughly, fully, through and through)

and stayed up with her that night, resonating comfort and feeling her pain as if it were my very own. The priest, a man of the cloth, God's ordained substitute, had

> deemed her gentle selfless soul unworthy,
>   destined for hell,
>   or at best perennial purgatory.

And all the while he never recognized her most gentle and soulful side.

Medicine Wheel 1987

Still wearing the blue feather tucked behind my ear, I hiked back up the short hill from picnic table to campfire. We were happy, contented, and exhausted from our day; our voices in soft dulcet tones that evening while we took turns roasting marshmallows on sticks. At evening's end and when the campfire reduced once again to coal embers, we said our good nights and all turned in early. The next day we would each be on our own to meditate, hike, or talk or read or snooze. When I returned to my cabin once again, I anchored the quill of the blue feather under my clock and crawled into bed to read. Within minutes, I turned the reading lamp off, dropped the book by my side and placed my glasses, as usual, carefully on the floor where I could easily get to them. I fell asleep quickly that night, lulled by the deepening quiet and background choir of river and insect night songs that wafted through the narrowly opened screened window.

BAM!

Startled with a sudden bang at the door, I bolted straight up, suddenly fully alert and sitting straight up where moments before I had been lying, curled warmly in a delicious dreamless sleep. I quickly swiveled my legs and sat on the edge of the bed and stared, confused, for a moment or two at the heavy wooden cabin door from where the sound had come.

Knock-knock.

Two sharp raps on the door. Maybe Erin or Janis couldn't sleep and just wanted to talk? Or maybe the baby was sick, or the bee-stings had turned ugly and someone needed a drive to the hospital?

I called out, "Hey!?" but got no answer. I wasn't concerned for my safety at all, not there and not then. It was just us in the immediate area; we had more or less taken over that campsite area for the weekend. I got up out of bed and walked over to the heavy wooden door and questioned once more, a bit louder this time.

"HEY!?" I called out again.

But still no answer, only the continuous droning of the night sounds responded through the open window that faced the river. But the door faced the deep woods and led out onto a simple decked porch. Perhaps the visitor could not hear me call out through the thick pine walls? More curious than anything, I unlatched the door and slowly swung its heavy mass out a few inches, and took a good look. No one was there! Just the empty porch, well illuminated by the overhead light. I had a clear view of the area and listened acutely. Definitely, definitely, no one was there. I felt it and I knew it.

Laughing a bit to myself (self-consciously as usual), more as a release of tension than apprehending anything really funny about the situation, I again swung the door shut and re-latched it. Now what was that all about? I did get awakened by a heavy bang and did hear a knocking at the door about a minute before. I was suddenly fully awake, the brush of night air through the open door had indeed shaken off any remaining residue of sleep. I walked over to the little picnic table in the room under the window and popped the top off my Lil' Coleman ice chest. Tipping the jug of grapefruit juice to my lips, I glanced over at the clock on the other side of the room and realized that I did not have my glasses on.

Artist Musings

It was at that moment of realization that
I saw what I saw,
felt what I felt,
and *knew*
life is much more than a sequence of unrelated dots, notes, events.

Something of a shiver and chill moved right through me in the room, then a sparkle flash something caught my eyes and I knew, just Knew, from the direction of the flow, that whatever had just moved through me was now floating directly in front of me.

A huge mass of swirling, scintillating, silvery-blue points of light
 danced only five to seven inches in front and slightly above me—
  a most incredible fireworks display!
   Hundreds of them, teeny-tiny atoms of light,
    each dancing to its own rhythms
     and weaving and reweaving glittersparkles across the gossamer web that connected the whole form,
      a form that was vaguely round,
       then shifting to oval,
       and then back to

round and so on,
over and over.
But, oh! the depth, too!
It was animated. It was alive!
It was loving words and tender touches,
it was newly welcoming and an ancient old friend. It was one and more than one—
a family—an essence I belonged with.

They had come to collect me, remind me to re-collect myself with Us. Literally, they had knocked on the door and I had answered.

Swirls within swirls,
at faster than speed-of-light speeds,
the points of light flashed and shimmered.
The silvery-blues wove into a wispy web;
the constantly moving points of light became sparkled
with fourteen-carat gold and ultraviolet pulses,
some flashes of rose and deep forest green.
And of course, an overlay of that dazzling bluefeather
and bluestar and butterfly-wing cosmic color
that always had, and would forever, resonate deep within me.

We shared a good laugh too, that swirling mass of lights and me.
(I was grateful that it visited within

inches of my face,
> so I could see with my eyes as well as my being.).

Knowledge, ageless wisdom, perennial truths conveyed,
> communicated, infused into every cell of my being,
>> all in a momentary *Flash!*

Some understood immediately and some stored away for future animation, like acorn nuts that rest dormant until it is suddenly their time to burst forth and grow.

> (When it would be my time to Know.)

I knew that it would take a lifetime to unfold and evolve its secrets. That, too, was major part of the message and it rang loud and clear, propelled on a phosphorescent streaming beam of silver blue light.

Then,
> one by one the lights blinked out.
> And, I was left standing,
>> just staring,
>>> at a pair of pale yellow dime-store curtains fluttering in the night breeze before me.

I tumbled back into bed and tried to recover what I could, anchor it into anything that I knew or had heard before that could help me understand, make sense out of something that literally made no sense. Somehow, I drifted off to a deep sleep. Only when sunlight streamers filled my cabin, and the morning birds were well into their daily songs, did I awaken.

Medicine Wheel 1987

Normally a very early riser, I discovered with a start that I had slept late into that next morning. I was still full of questions, as well as a bit dazed about the door knocks and giving entry to something that was beyond anything my rational mind could "figure out." The sun had already moved into mid-morning time, and breakfast had come and gone. We gathered on Janis' porch to plan our day as Bob strummed guitar chords along in the background. The baby gurgled away, contented to just sit in his day chair batting his spoon in rhythm and counterpoint to the voices and music surrounding him.

We were in for another scorcher of a day with record high humidity. But for that mid-morning, it was still clear and fresh among in the forests of the Blue Hills. The warm breezes fanned overhead and reshuffled the grand old trees above, while the Tye River glistened and sparkled, lazy in its late summer pace, but nonetheless continuing as always to move purposely toward its destination.

I don't recall how much detail I gave the group that morning about my encounter with the blue-light special. Probably very little, knowing me and knowing my preference to hold on to information until I can better explain or understand. That experience was not one that I understood and I really didn't have the words to explain, if I even do today. I did, however, ask the group if anyone had knocked on my door in the middle of the night. Casual shakes of heads and a chorus of "No's" and "nuh-uh's" to that question reassured me that there were no practical jokers in the bunch. Most didn't even raise an eyebrow to the question. Janis asked why I asked, and I simply said that I had thought I heard a loud bang and then a knock on my door around 1:30 a.m., but more shakes of heads convinced me that they had no clue. Their painful bee-stings had begun to turn into itchy stings, and it was all they could do to just concentrate on not scratching and plan some languid activities for the day.

We planned to meet around noon, when the sun was high overhead, and cross the river one more time to the Wheel together. The magnificent multifaceted quartz that had been placed so reverently the day before would then be removed in silent ceremony. The remaining stones of the wheel would stay, intact, hidden well away on the far side of the river in the depths of that ancient forest. Our contribution to the Harmonic Convergence would then be officially closed that Sunday afternoon.

Until then we were on our own, and I desperately needed some time to reflect and assimilate what had gone on the day and night before. Indeed, what had gone on? Silvery blue swirls in the air above my head, a rush through my body, a knock at the door that I had answered. Some formless shape of a message (an infusion) and some gentle laughter shared. Not a lot to begin with, but maybe if I worked at it long enough, I could logically figure it out.

One other curious note to this tale, however, was the fate of the blue feather. The girls noticed immediately that I was not wearing it that morning. It was not tucked behind my ear or being carried around like the day before. In my haste to get up, get out, and get on with the program, I had forgotten to grab it on my way out the cabin door. Yet when I went back into my cabin to retrieve it, it was not under the clock where I had left it the night before. In fact, I turned that small square room upside down in my search for *my* feather. It was nowhere to be found! Nowhere! I knew that I had secured it under the clock the night before. That particular feather was important to me, a memento of sorts that represented the whole weekend. I looked everywhere, and nowhere was there my special blue feather. Having no clue to solve *this* latest mystery, I latched the cabin door and walked out to the grounds to tell my friends. I must have looked like someone who had lost her best friend; but then, that is how I felt. Amid encouraging words like "don't worry, you'll find it" and "it was only meant for you to have on the wheel building day" and so on, I walked over to my car parked in the clearing. One of the young women moving to Santa Fe and I had planned to take a hike up to the lower circuit of the Falls that morning.

I was amazed that the lower Crabtree Falls was such a short drive! It was just over the next hill – surprisingly close to where we were staying. Before that weekend, I had always reached the Falls from the upper mountain ridge side and never driven *up from the valley* before. I filed this geographic relationship away for future use. Someday it might be important, come in handy, as indeed it would eleven years later when I stood on butterfly-tree island and gazed *down* river. But for then, eleven years before, a short morning hike was perfect, and we hiked with mid-morning gusto *up* to the mother boulder that overlooked the lower level of the Falls. Neither of us was interested in continuing several hours' climb that would switch back and wind up to the upper ridge of the Falls. We both crawled onto that huge sightseeing rock that under-looked the lower plunging Falls and simply sat, peaceful and contented, hypnotized by the patterns of water that tumbled over the rock ledge directly in front of us.

      She told me about Gaia, the Earth Mother theory, that day. This new friend of friends had a way of telling Gaia's story that made Her come alive to me. That area of the Blue Hills would continue to live on within me, etched deeply into my mind, body, and soul—forever associated with the enduring resourcefulness, depths of our earthly home, the knock at the cabin door, and the infusion of swirling lights of information.

Medicine Wheel 1987

Back in my cabin after our hike, it was time to return to my apartment in Richmond and to the business end, the other side, of Life's great divide. I quickly packed my bag, emptied the water from the cooler, then turned to strip the sheets off of the bed.

Flutter, flutter, fly!

Out popped my blue feather, evidently lodged at the very foot of the bed between the sheets! I watched as it floated for a couple of seconds, simply wafting and turning in the air, before landing on the hard yellow pine floor. With a grin, I picked it up and twirled it in my fingers in amazement. My "friend" was back! How, when, what the...huh? Questions asked with no answers. But I knew this: Just as that blue feather had greeted me when I first arrived, it would be with me on my return drive home. And most importantly, it had been with me throughout the vision, creation, building and the ceremony of our medicine wheel. I laughed with joy at the exquisite timing and beauty of it all. And as I laughed, I heard and felt, once again, those melodies of delighted laughter, both beyond me and sweeping through me.

Haunting Melody

We would leave Los Angeles spiritually bankrupt. Dad would bark and Mom would cry, I would endure appendicitis and my sister would hold tea parties with her imaginary friend. In the Spring of 1963, my appendicitis came on swiftly. Dad diagnosed and treated me with strict bed-rest (perhaps some homemade antibiotic...he said that bread-mold penicillin saved his life and leg back in the war).

>>> No doctors, however, not even a house call
>>>> if they even conducted house calls there
>>>>> in that strange overflowing
>>>> metropolis of L.A.
>>>>>> (where Watts nearby
>>>>> would blow up to
>>>>>>> burn baby burn
>>>>>> two summers later...
>>>>>>>> just before
>>>>>>> we moved
>>>>>>>>> to
>>>>>>>> the Desert
>>>>>>>> SW).

Meanwhile, back in the apartment, I was burning, baby, burning with fever again. The appendix threatened to burst, and all the while Dad was saying that if I didn't get better, *he* would conduct the surgery

>> (he had done it once before on a ship,
> he announced).

Oh great! And what was he going to use for anesthesia — beer or whiskey? The cure sounded worse than the malady and I willed myself better. Collectively, we had an aversion to doctors and hospitals, medications and medical bills. Strange, isn't it, for all the training and lessons and connections with the medical field, they elected less, not more contact with it. Talk about survival do-it-yourselfers!

Well, anyway, I got better slowly but surely. That late Spring when the fifth grade came to the end, I read the commencement speech but was not allowed to march in the May parade.

By then, when
    we moved to the desert,
        the edge of Death Valley to be
more exact,
    Mom was beside herself,
        uprooted once again
        while Dad tried to hold down the fort
    wherever Life took us.

For us, the geography and weathers of each location were as different as night and day. Such a range of extremes of land forms and emotional climates spanning from the lush watered evergreens, amphibious frogs, and garden snakes of the Pacific NW to the Yucca trees, horny toads, and rattling sidewinders of the SW sands of desert China Lake

.

(We needed a special pass to get through *that* gate.)

A riddle: How come there was a Naval Base smack dab in the middle of the desert, on a lakebed long forgotten in geologic time? Once or twice a year when we folk-dancers did our rain dance, or humidity happened with just a few fleeting fluffy clouds in the sky, the outer weather would change. But the inner emotional climate? It silently raged, stormed, and we wept buckets of fresh and salty tears.

Needless to say, Mom did not thrive in the desert. We lived in two houses there. She was like a fish out of water, gasping in the dry desert air, talking to the couple of neighbor ladies who also had children. Rather than sharing literature, the women would sagely share recipes and the latest in potty training gleaned from Dr. Benjamin Spock's book of the day. A trip to the country club was a treat for her—time-out for a swim and a martini (or few), needed to hold herself together, under the glowing tiki-tiki lights.

We kids, of course, took like fish to water in the Olympic-sized swimming pool. That summer, the country club became my oasis for fun and play, which included French fries with extra ketchup, sunbathing, giggling with girlfriends and playing numerous games of chess.

> I had learned chess in the South Gate of L.A.
> (for once I was twelve,
> I was old enough to see it more
> than checkered moves).

I enjoyed a game here and there with a young sexy foreign engineer during visits to the pool. I was fourteen going on eighteen and chess was all we played, but what fun to learn the names of the pieces in another language, hear a different accent. Oh, what a delicious crush I had on him that summer! Kiddie competitions of summer vacation chess would never be the same! Chess was one bright spot in the midst of the silent stormy home life, as were my school friends, international folk dancers, and fellow musicians from the school orchestra. Treasures they were to me, each one of them, for they were my oases, my centers of sanctuary amidst the hurricane storms of home and youthful hormones.

Blue Hills Diary

PART III: INFUSED BY SKY AND EARTH

Meditation

I draw a circle around myself and hold precious inner thoughts. Complete stillness surrounds me and I am aligned in perfect peace, choosing only to observe Nature's first rustles of lazy awakening on this new day. I enter the courtyard and am not noticed, nor do I alert others as they go about their morning business.

As I stepped out of the car onto the parking lot, I felt such supreme solitude. As my left < boot touched the pavement, I immediately began to sense myself expanding, lightening up for the rush of it all; the luxury of unlimited time. By the time I had walked around to the boot of the car, to leisurely exchange my pocketbook for a light jacket, I knew also that this bubble of no particular time and no particular place was perfect. Everything was perfectly in synch, perfectly aligned, perfectly harmonized and in tune with what had been created for and by my desire. This I knew—that I had somehow discovered a particular door, a way station, where there would be no interruptions that morning. I had found a safe pal of time and space that would embrace and protect me. I felt at peace and at home.

I tied the arms of the jacket around my waist, plus double-checked to make sure that my keys were safely secured, squared away in the depths of one of the pockets. All this before locking the car and taking leave of the well traveled paved rood of the parking area. I decided not to take the sketchbook this time around after all and left it in the car instead. Rather, I desired to capture the exquisite silence, the brilliant radiant colors of the rising day (star) and experience (sense) adventures as they came. After all, I would need to get back into my (body) car again! Crabtree Park—Procrustean indeed!

Half Moon Bridge revisited

The half moon bridge beckoned me forward, onward to the other, far side of the Tye River. The little path to the bridge wove a trail of deliciously fragrant wildflower and herb aromas spawned at the height of summer. All of nature was abloom that late summer with her luxuriant growth along the river. As I meandered along to the bridge, abundant flora riches reached out to me, twining along both sides of the little narrow path, seeming eager to pollinate my sneakers, pant legs, jacketed hips, shoulders and hair when I brushed by them. Alongside on the left <, the river's waters playfully splashed over the stones, offering harps of happy gurgling sounds in rhythm and tempo to my sauntering pace.

To salute this bright new day, I desired once again to cross over that particular stone and wood bridge that rose symmetrically above the river. Then I would have precious time (all time) to energetically hike back up to the first level of the Falls, before finally accepting the butterflies' invitation to visit their island by mid-morning. The damp floral aromas, the piney air, I savored and inhaled deeply with such gratitude for our continued life and health. I had returned to my sacred place! Her siren's song had called me back to her over and over, over the years, and for the past few weeks and last days her call had risen intensely just prior to my arrival. A call and an invitation I could no longer ignore.

How lucky I was to have the ability and the capacity to move at will, to drink in with all my full functioning senses the sensual delights around me! In that sudden burst of realization (and revelation), I celebrated these knowings and gave thanks to Aurora's rising sun that morning at the apex of the bridge. What a gift! This new day with her river, the rocks, the trees, the scrub, and the butterfly-tree island that was just beginning to shimmer and come to life in the light of life before me. And most of all, I gave thanks to and felt profound gratitude for the people I love, have loved, and who have loved me over my years of this life on earth.

I sealed my prayer and connected with the hearts of all that I could touch as I stretched, balanced in movements of my own Tai-Chi design, faced fully the sun and joyfully greeted the morning and the four points at the midpoint of half moon bridge.

An Aside

That morning's insight (receiving requested solitude) was quite a jolt of epiphany. There would be many others that day, and for times to come, each a little more personally stunning than those before. As I revisit these words once again months later, I can approach, retrospectively, whole patterns of interactions that took place over those two days. These, in turn, continue to *unfurl* and join with other similar patterns of exceptional experience that have taken place over my lifetime. These Blue Hills always seamed for me (seemed to me) an almost magnetic pull (together) of the myriad mystical experiences that have been ineffable, impossible to explain before.

Too, many more individuals are connecting these days; recognizing, remembering, and sharing their experiences. As our human web connects across the network, we share the fun *unfurl*ing these mysteries together. My story is only one, often a lonely one, but I offer my words with myriad meanings nonetheless. Sense what resonates with you, contemplate and add more of your own (now won) meanings.

> (Perhaps we all can discover the words
> to express our experiences together.)

Unfurl

To simply put it into words:
When we let go of our human need to control time and events
—when we trust and surrender our little will's design and desires—
then we align ourselves to the Universal Matrix
(we-eve)
of time sequencing and space placing.
What we set out and send out in our desire is what we align;
What we receive is our perceived answer.
Answer is created from the confluence of intense desire,
Between personal and universal will to be
(overlap that)
what manifests in form.
What manifests in form—formulates formally and informs—
is called an event, an actualized point connected,
co-created and formed within Matrix—
our Mother of infinite possibilities, potentials and forms.
The More (overlaps) avenues we have with Matrix,
the more we attune,
harmonize,
sing to The One song—
Universe—we all share.

An Aside

At this point in writing this account, my rational mind and sense of self- protection are sending up red flags: "Be careful; you'll seem crazy!" Did you *really* want to say these words and go in that direction? Are you *sure* you want to continue this way? Will you sacrifice all that you have built professionally and academically over your lifetime just to tell a story? It will only get weirder as you continue... warning, warning!

It took several days in 1998 to return to this diary and continue.

Artist Musings

I eagerly began my hike that second day, up to the lower levels of the Falls again. The sun moved in rhythm to the breezes of the trees canopied overhead.

>Sparkling glimmers of contrasting bright and shadow onto my path
>>and over as the river flowed downstream
>>>to its Source
>>>>and I trudged uphill
>>>>>in counterpoint alongside.

The world around me smelled delicious—
>sweet, green and new from sassafras, pine, and the morning dew
>>and yet, the overriding aroma of overripe vegetation and earth
>>>reminded me that the Autumn was not far away.

The profound silence, and paradoxically the sounds of breezes
>sweeping lazily through the trees in waves
>>and the river pulsing alongside in rhythm
>>>as it filled, lapped, giggled, and flowed
>>>>over and around the boulders.

My footsteps, heartbeat and deep breathing,
>keeping pace with those eternal and internal rhythms.

I recalled the Dance
 that had been forgotten
 in my hectic days back
home.

Hike into Infinity

 Once again I was intimately, integrally
connected with and drawn into the magic space
surrounding me and rising inside of me; sensing deeply
that at that moment and in that place it was essential
for me to *Be*. I Knew that it was just as essential for
me to be there, then, as it was for any other of Nature's
expressions I was observing.

 My footsteps pounding the Earth,
 my breath exchanging the air,
 my arms pumping breezes of
 their own to shift
 the leaves reaching out
 into the path as I passed
 were essential,
 as was the heat radiating
 and salty sweat produced from
 my body's workout
 and the wonder and profound
 gratitude I felt in my soul.

 All essential, all necessary, all in dynamic
 phase and in perfect balance
 with the Great Spirit who had called me to *be*
 traveling there and then.

 With each step I took, I knew that I was
retracing steps that I had taken many times before *and*

simultaneously forging, releasing new ones to follow yet again for another time.

Flashes of bygone memories became alive and I sighed with recognition, perfect contentment and deep understanding as my awareness gathered wings and grew. To come to (become) awareness of my essential, unique *signature* upon this place and time, to knowing deeply inside, to understand and stand under my journey there and then was necessary to *Life* as She and we and each of us (no difference) continue to create and express ourselves.

This awareness made me feel infinitely great and small at the same time:
> That somehow, in some way, my essence, my personal signature was vital there and then to assist with
>> our together universal grand design and masterpiece.

That surprise, that moment of insight, was tremendously humbling and steeped deep and rich with the awesome interconnections of our choices, our alignments and potent with meaning. To answer the "Call" when it comes, and our willingness and timeliness to call backwards and forward until we catch each other in tune. To discover in our short or long distance our mutual connection, our communication, our communion.

I had been called to do my part and my part had always been and would forever be just what was needed,
> *whether I was conscious of it or not.*

On that morning, I once again re-membered, fully conscious, aware of *IT*
>
> while layers and layers of design, purpose, and meaningfulness
>
>> *unfurl*ed, unfolded, and whispered their secrets to me
>>
>>> this gift of Love—the calling to remembrance—
>>>
>>>> visited me that day while during my hike
>>>>
>>>>> up and down one generous, gracious,
>>>>>
>>>>>> blooming Blue Hill.

Unfurl

Pieces of the puzzle, discovered from—
formed completely by (eye!) and our now own won (ow!) clues.
Limited sequences perceived of (non) random
shuffling of vision and pain,
such is our lot in life that ties us
tightly into our limitations.

Yet, could my involved story be similar to yours, and together our story continue?
Backwards, forwards, and inside out—
our inscendences grant us our transcendences.

The fragments and prisms of ourselves in search of Mysteries
(meld) together as they unfold.

A paradox, yes.
One that grants
—pleases us with (glimpses) a wholly conscious death, resurrection—
bestows our salvation.

(Human nature as it is.)
No longer an ambiguous duality parade of two by two.
But twos aligned together (duets)
creating octaves of harmonies

*singing More than the
sum of their parts.
(1+1 >2).
Human nature too, to honor singular
manifestations into forms
(such as "I") to construct in tandem
our multidimensional net we
weave throughout between us.
One that has been designated and time-date
stamped
by our common five senses
hence limited to our shared
human bond
of perceived limitations; the
contemporary rules of time and space.
Those images we (seek you) and me via
imagination avenue
are our unique powers (doubled) to
initiate new worlds;

and
born we are of different drummers and
brilliant prisms (leitmotifs).
Yet, together we gather (unique),
in resonance, in sequence, our net—
continuously folding and
unfolding,
and evolving—
Homeward bound once
again.*

Harmonic Note

Friend Phil asked me one day, "Are you from this planet?"

I replied with a quip, "Of course, aren't we all? It has just been a long adjustment period."

An Aside

I felt totally humbled that my ongoing study and questing into the mysteries of synchronicity had been given new dimensions rising above the worn-out mantras of, "There are no accidents" and, "Carl Jung coined the term synchronicity to describe...." Many folks from all walks of life are, and certainly I am, tantalized by synchronicity's profundity, its greater mystery, and so we pursue its essential meaning that, paradoxically, always seems to lie just out of reach when clutched too vigorously. Yet as we extract personal meaningfulness from each one we experience, over a lifetime they begin to share their secrets *if* we follow their threads *and* begin to weave our life's tapestry into the greater *tapestry* of All-Life.

So, in sewing and as my greater awareness gathered
and dawned on that mountainside that morning
    and I centered myself to still point,
        I suddenly realized with profound clarity
           the multidimensional *meaning*
           and role of synchronicity
                as it converged on, within
           and through me.
Like a sudden, orgasmic bolt of lightning,

tremendous insight and clarity filled my bodymind and soul,
> grounding my feet deeply into the core of the Mother Earth.

While simultaneously, the top of my head blasted out and up
> like a beacon of Light into the far reaches of the sky above me.

>> (Perfectly aligned,
>> perfectly in phase)
> the Light that flowed through me on that vertical plan high and low
>> stretched from core to sky,
> extended as far as I could only (then) imagine
>> with my limited mind,
>>> but could vitally *feel* "clicking" contact with

(aligning, seeking, being in alignment with - pick one –

>>> it is indescribable
>> with only words)
>> an infinite series of Phases, Sources, Intelligences.

Ancient Melody

One day (it might have been early Spring or Autumn ...the sky was moderately cloudy; the air a bit brisk) when Mae and I were little ones skipping along the sidewalk to Wing's grocery store, I froze in mid-skip, stunned. This very distant childhood memory still haunts me today, and it takes considerable effort to pull, or should I say tug, it forward from the recesses of my mind. Now, as this journal continues to cover well into my 48th year, well over one year has passed since I began again to write to solve the riddle of that day in 1957.

It was a most demanding exceptional experience that seamed to cross into no man's land between the realms of
     mystical, encounter, and psi *
                                *sigh

[*the 23rd letter of the Greek alphabet,
     scribed like Neptune's trident of the unknown]

Now, the Wing's was a mom and pop grocery
     (as was the Steinman's store in the other direction
          two blocks up and one over, or, was it the other way around?
              Regardless, it was the Knight's move of geography.)

But that day, with Mae, we girls were eager to go straightaway to Wing's store to pick up the few items our mothers had requested and to spend a couple of pennies on candy.

> (The Wing family always let us walk behind the counter to inspect and select the latest treats. The two for one candies were a special deal for us, as were the
> Smith's Brothers cough drops (@ five cents a box—
> medicine not candy—Mom would scold).

So, skipping along in a southeasterly direction all of a sudden,
    that feeling of whooosh!
        I stopped, Mae stopped, we stopped mid-skip in time and
            The silent sound... continues and booms...

            In fusion!
            Remember!
                Who you
            are!
            Why you are!

I replied, to nobody in particular, ...
    er,
        ah,
            well, now,
    ain't this a turnaround of events.
The moment lasted forever
    (until it was at last completed)
        and when over,
            I stood solidly back on the sidewalk staring around, uncertain of my surroundings...
oh yeah,

okay,
>> uhuh,
>>>> ayep,
>>>>>> yes, indeedy.

I was my old self, set back in place and time, again.

The crater of dug out soil to my right in a neighbor's yard was where we kids would run up and down for hours some days, just loving that incline. It makes me smile today to catch these words and this feeling, particularly when recalling that silent and booming voice. That day, Mae and I were left < spinning, then standing dumbstruck in mid skip to Wing's under that brighter than overcast day.

After the infusion, and once that voice had spoken, I stopped spinning, and asked Mae point blank: Do you ever feel like you are the only [human conscious] being and everyone else is er, ummmm, like "not-real" around you?

She replied: No, can't say that I do. But her crystal blue eyes betrayed her; they were still a bit wild-looking. She looked at me with fear and that look, then threw a thought back to me that I caught from earlier childhood experiences and recognized well:

Putty, are you crazy?
>> Silly Putty me, (my nickname on the islands), you goofed again.

I learned yet again that morning that I had gone to and spoken of a place where words of these far-out experiences are sometimes better left < unspoken, for they do not make it right > for another.

Best to just avoid the subject of
weird stuff.
And as that moment came and went,
who could say what it was or
what it meant
(but I had an inkling of my blueprint
inking that day).
Afterwards, life continued as life does, and did,
and Mae and I never spoke again of that
flash zap in-fusion
(from above ^ in front: and to the
> from < field)

The remainder of that day and visit to the
Wing's store is a relative blank in my mind these days,
with only fragments of flashbacks of an infusion at that
moment that traveled through the mirrors of time and
recall, caught today only in my retrospective looking
glass of reverie.

When I step back into that time (via imagination
and/or memory... who knows?), My reaction early on
to that intensity becomes a river of questions beginning
with:
Why was the "I" in this, me body?
Who were the other i's in their own
(separate) me bodies?
Was Mae an I
or a me?
Was she real or not, perhaps a robot
(although she sure
seemed real enough to
me).

Even a couple of discrete questions, posed well over thirty years later to a psychologist friend, yielded no solid answers. These types of questions and those in-depth studies of psychology (the beginnings of often frantic efforts) to make sense of seemingly bizarre out of the "norm" events were and are the very real experiences of life. These and those, and our experiences that have remained hidden, lost, forgotten, or bypassed and feared by general society.

But in truth, that day, this five-year-old child had been zapped somehow in some way. And something within me changed that would linger as questions and follow me for years to come.

(I still sense the craft overhead, the lighter brighter sky, in the southeast that day,
    and that constellation of discovery would not be any less monumental
               than the times spent in the Blue
        Hills,
                 I write to you today.)
    Say what you will, and be comfortable with your own resonance.
        For the gift is to ask Why?
            And wonder with the deepest
       wonder and awe.

My wonder, my questions that morning then as now when the spinning stopped, was why I was me, who was I, and whether other people and beings shared the same I Am that I Am. That perhaps we are filled with something (Spirit and Mind) into our different vessels, human formed bodies, we each call "me." Or rationally thinking, we are just at that age becoming aware of each, our own consciousness... consciousness being first aware of itself? A conundrum, born that day, still reverberating.

>Otherwise, why am I not (also) in the body of another,
>>a friend or
>>>a dog or a goat, or
>>>>a cat or a horse?
>>>>>Why not a stone
>>>>>or a cabbage in the field?
>>>>>>Indeed,
>>>>>>why not butterfly?

Harmonic Note

The ancient Mayans said the answer simply in their greetings:
>In Lake'ch.
>To translate: *I am another yourself.*

Unfurl

Holy Mother of the Universe,
can you even begin to imagine my surprise
when the Light that I was
conducting through me
from deepest cores to
reaches unknown
was being
acknowledged
and
echoed
back to in-form
me?
At that very moment
I simply
understood
(and stood under and
over and inside the Light).

I would never (again) forget how essential we humans are to convey, transform and transmute information as that Light that
streams
faster than the
speed of Light
and to communicate other
consciousnesses, intelligences
of Universe via particle dots and wave dashes
both together in digital and analog, both and
more absolutely necessary those fuzzy sets to
set order out of chaos by intent and desire.

No Time, simply relative speed
measures to Be—

*a lifetime of synchronistic
patterns,*
*lifetimes of recollection,
and choices
made along the
way merged—*
*all
together at
Once.
My quest and prayer for understanding
my role
and reason for the calling to this
place at that moment
(timeless time, placeless
place) had been answered.*

*I wept from my depths, my remembering place,
for the exquisite joy and in gratitude,
for the flood had finally burst
forth—
those dead, buried
emotions—and
reconnection,
discovery, and
awareness.*

*Still lightening struck and beaming the warmth of light
inside and through me,
I fairly flew back down the mountainside, finally
ready, eager to connect
with whatever awaited me More
that day—
the beckoning embrace
of those butterfly trees.*

Synergy

I breathe deeply to resonate with the music of complementary energy surrounding me. To discover that all consciousness was necessary to the formulation of that moment—that we had converged to gather at point in that particularly time and place. I hold the moment close to my heart as we align and we dance together in celebration, in the gardens between heaven and earth.

Filled with tremendous awe and ecstatic joy for the zapping bolt above and below and from out of the blue, I paid particular attention to retrace my footsteps back down the mountainside. Still in a place of realization of conscious interconnection, I gave thanks to all of the rocks, knotted roots, twists, turns and encroaching trees that had formed my path up the mountain just moments and eons earlier. Already, the warming morning sun was rising, spreading light streams through the grand old trees, and had awakened the swarms of gnats and other flying critters, in search of my salt and heated flesh.

More than anything else, I *knew* and had *discovered* that I was essential to this place, to this time, and had been called there then to loop and intersect one small cycle of my own with some greater cycle of which I was needed, necessary, and fully integral.

> And, that my part in this never ending drama of creation and transformation
> had in *one* perfect moment of still-point balance,
> speaking without words

                    of
Alignment,
            harmonic resonance that
                ripplewaved and
                        swept across an infinite
                    series of intersecting cycles
                            into the deepest
                        and farthest reaches of
                                inner and
                                outer
                                space and
                                time.

    My magic mountain area had called me and had I listened to Her call, all the while thinking that it was *my* need that I was following. It was, "of course," as we would speak of the river's course. And, coincidentally in following and attuning to my own need, my call, I caught the deeper insights of synchronicity, in a matrix of the Mother Nature of meaning and Her continuously woven and weaving tapestry. How absolutely humbling and empowering at the same time!

    To grasp and insight that even the tiniest, most inconsequential, and yes, even the most thoughtless of actions and intents
            re-weaves the greater Weave
                    and has the power to recall the
Weaver.

    As I slowed down to re-cross and then finally stop at the middle of the half moon bridge, I gazed out onto the Tye River once again and quickly located the butterfly trees. Now fully illuminated and spotlighted by the rising sun, they were already alive and teeming with activity. The iridescent blues were again most abundant. Scores of them, floating on the river's updraft and swaying, with the gentle breezes that continued to flow in warming currents between the rocky shores.

    En masse, seen from a distance, they shimmered,
        reflecting shadings of peacock, royal, and ultraviolet blue.
    Their sunshine dance a delight, swaying in tandem and in pulse alight
        and awash against the shadowy background
            of the deeper fir trees above and meadow green bushes
        with their golden orange honeyed fragrance to the nose
        and rocky-thorns of ground shrubs to our landing feet
            invitation and re-entry for me
                into their
            everyday world.

An Aside

A funny thing, perspective. As I gazed at the butterflies, I wondered about those whom over my lifetime had gazed at me in much the same way, from a more distant vista.

Were my activities in the daily tasks of busyness as localized, as limited as swarming around the area of my birth never to really leave that area until I died? Rhetorically speaking anyway? Certainly I had moved away from the place of my birth by the time I was a toddler and by sweet sixteen had lived far away, on the opposite coast, from where I had spent my early childhood years. Too, I have by now already lived in nine states and twenty-four different houses, the one today being the one home that I have lived in the longest—for over six years.

>(But the area we live in—
>or are called to—is not just
>restricted to a geographical location.)

Although these changes in residence were perhaps the most easily observable, my life has also been marked by shifting areas in other ways. Intellectual interests, career paths, friends, partners, and philosophical beliefs had all shifted, had *moved me* in some way over my lifetime. When I take a wide-angled perspective in space and time, I would say that one predominate feature, (indeed my signature and call to Life) has been highlighted by continued exploration, restless movement and motivated by some inner calling to discover new "locales." The source and the reason for that desire had always been a bit out of reach. Similar to the Tantalus, these experiences were just enough to tantalize me, keep me going, exploring, traveling, but not enough to really understand where all this activity was leading, much less what any major life theme and obvious road signs were apparent.

But even that realization was enough to really get me wondering and questioning, again after a long dry spell. I sympathized with the Tye River Valley those days, for we were both drained dry and needed some rejuvenating waters to replenish our flow. And in that wonder and heartfelt quest, that calling to return, *in that moment of knowing* on the mountainside, the revitalizing waters began once again to pour forth.

On another hand, no wonder I felt such a great sympathy, a sisterhood with those few iridescent blues who flew far afield from the safety, predictability, and security of the swarm.

They were mirrors of me!

And I just happened upon this seemingly "rare chance" of a lifetime to gaze into the mirror they offered that day, and discovered that it was reflected back to me in the brilliance of their butterfly wings. Those few explorers, those travelers, reached out to me, a foreigner to their world. It was time to have a closer look and walk through their mirror.

So it was on that mid-morning, a late summer's day, when I could no longer refuse their invitation. The circumstances which had led me to this moment (and I had reverently followed) were all pointing to this, their, invitation. I no longer had the excuses of self-consciousness, a frenzied schedule, or no time. I had been in-formed on the mountain and was wholly ready to receive and understand more of Life's teachings than ever before. It was a chance of a lifetime, a special gift, and I seized the moment while it hovered and scintillated around me.

The Explorer

With every step I took, every step of the way that I walked toward that path to the riverbank, my heart reached out in gratitude for this moment. I was acutely aware of the Light still within me, infused just a moment before (or was it lifetimes before?) on the Crabtree Falls mountainside. And thankfully, even the quality of that Light had shifted and I began to *know* as revealed through her many faces, her many qualities. No longer electrically charging me, zapping me, fused in place between Earth's inner core and the reaches of outer space, pulsing with each wave of in-formation received, I softened. As I walked (floated) over to the rocky shore and stepped between the open canopy of the overhanging trees, all was peace, supreme contentment, and I felt a deep settling inside of me.

>
> With exquisite realization,
> > I knew that I was being
> > > introduced to Light's
> > personalities, her many dimensions, octaves, harmonic resonances, intelligences, consciousnesses, and faces,
> > > and each one conveyed its own
> > distinctive quality.

Now, instead of the nuclear blast of pulsing waves,

Light once again shifted and showed another face.

She was sublime—centered, muted, and softly conveying a warm golden glow perfectly matched and aligned with all of the tones, the tranquility and raw, natural beauty surrounding me.

Rhapsody

    Oh, my dears! Had anyone ever, ever felt so blessed as this? My heart sang with joy and that joy transmuted as yet into another form of Light radiating out in all directions, connecting time and place with the glue of love and gratitude for the remembered and forgotten people, places, and events that had shaped my life.

    And remarkably, that love and gratitude echoed back into my heart, no one, no place, and no event forgotten.
    All bonded together—*we were*—communing
        one to One;
            heart to Heart;
                soul to Soul.

    No longer ecstatic as on the mountainside, I was instead linked in silent communion and in touch with all that echoed back to me.

        (How long we communed like this, I do not know.)

The faces I have worn in my life, and yes, those shape-shifted over "lifetimes"
    communicated with the many different faces, voices, consciousnesses

            (and paradoxically many to a
        singular conduit)

                of Light we
              fashioned between us.

My natural, unadorned, many-faces face over time and place was exposed for *All* to see. And simultaneously there they echoed back in Light for *me* to see. In a flash and over timeless ages, I saw the multitude,
and, in that moment, myselves gathered together and re-membered.

And, in that essential connection, I returned Home.

Continuing

When we examine the continuance of things, the natural tendencies of heaven and earth can be seen. Therein lies the secret of eternity....

Like a continuous filling and draining, each visit to this act of writing reveals more to write; to honor what has honored me and to somehow capture and bring to shore all the connections and insights that were spawned that late summer's morning. Through this creative act of writing, I bring forth fully yet again all the magic and wonder of those days, nothing seems lost and much continues to come together.

I am joyful to have captured my Ox
(member of the seen and unseen star constellation)
and finally be able to be bringing her Home—
the unseen and lost in between—
after decades of close encounters and near misses.

The sun sparkled off the tiny surface wavelets, reaching deeply into the channels of the mightily depleted Tye River. Still, unceasingly, her channels were fed by the waterfalls above, which then merged and divided, and continued to meet and gradually erode some of the massive boulders that stood in her way. I watched, for there was no frustration, no angry confrontation, between these inter-playing forces and gentles of nature. Rather, the elements, all five I observed, played their parts and combined as one in constant rhythm, moving in synchrony, and always in constant communion with one another. Each was essential, each necessary, needed and required. Otherwise, there would be no building up and breaking down, no interplay, no eternal rhythm, or perennial dance of life.

Without this balance, exchange and interplay, Life ceases to exist. And I realized that without my essential contribution to this, our daily dance, my life would cease to exist not only as I knew it, but also
      because my part in the grand pattern was
    necessary,
      needed,
          and required.
            RSVP, costumes
        optional.

The Boulder

    Firmly situated downstream (between half moon bridge and butterfly tree island) rested, sleeping, a huge slate-gray boulder. Casually thrown into the river by some playful child one distant day past, it was necessary for the creation of the island that that would follow.

    The foundation was composed of
        smaller rocks,
            sand and grit (it would take nine
            full years to get rid of it)
                the taller honeysuckle
            trees,
                    the dense newer
                scrub and grasses,
                    and the
                    sweet orange
                    flower nectar
                that fed and sustained
                the world of emerging
                      butterflies
each declaring its life cycle within a multitude of nested lifetime cycles.

    Like some half- forgotten child's nursery rhyme
        about meeting a man with seven wives
on the Road to St. Ives,
            I too, was part of the
            equation
            —and the answer to that riddle.

    I could choose to play the part of the detached observer or fully recognize my part in the drama

unfolding around me,
>>inviting me to join.
>Whether I chose to acknowledge my part or not, I knew
>>my Be-ing was essential to the ever folding and unfolding drama
>>>there and then, moving within and without me.
>Whatever I contributed, at whatever level of understanding, the honor of my wholly aware presence was required.

>My choice was simple:
>>Whether to join the party wearing a costumed mask or not.
>As best I could, I dropped my masks and costumes
>>>and stepped out from the near shore
>>>>onto the series of smaller rocks strewn
>>>>>pathwise, forming the bridge across
>the effervescent and splashing streamlets of late summer's Tye River.

>At midpoint, I eagerly climbed up onto the two or three foot high exposed surface of that massive rock that conveyed such newfound meaning to me. I took my position facing the rising sun, downstream toward recollection again, and met face to face with butterfly tree island.

>The boulder below me felt solid, deeply rooted in the riverbed and fed by the surrounding waters. She

embraced me securely and held me close to her sun-warmed breast like a mother. As during those days of the medicine wheel building, I always seemed to feel vertigo when stepping on rocks across water or climbing

>--and especially descending--
>>any sort of rocky cliff,
>>>but not this time.

This boulder rock was solid, secure.
>I was amazed at the ease in which I stepped across the smaller stones
>>and crawled onto her safe rocky perch.

An Aside

Where do these seemingly innate fears come from? They say that one of the baby's primal fears is that of falling. I think that is similar with other mammals too, but not sure at this point. For me, vertigo is not so much feeling dizzy as a fear of falling, losing my grip. (Now that is a point to ponder with all of its varieties of meanings!) Climbing up a ladder or a steep incline is not nearly as difficult for me as stepping back down again. When others run laughing down a steep hill, paying no mind to the chance of falling, I sit on my butt and scoot down rather than take a chance of rolling head over hills, er, heels. An Achilles heel at that!

To play with this thought for a while, I also am afraid of extreme speed or backing up in a car. Rather, I prefer to turn tightly, going backward and forward several times rather than take the chance of hitting another car, swinging wildly out (sight unseen) or oh!

The roller coasters are the worst!

To ride a roller coaster up and down with its wild aversion to gravity, catching just the angels (the angles) leaves me less than dead, and feeling limp and all spent out. Why *that* is a thrill to others, I have no clue. The Matterhorn Mountain at Disneyland roller coaster ride was one trial to last a lifetime.

(They had to carry me off that ride!)

And when descending steep stairs; my way is to take them slowly, easily: one step down < left, catch up > right, hold one-two, repeat as often as necessary. Not paying attention one morning, I tumbled down from a school chum's attic room, head over heels, and landed face down onto their kitchen floor. Illuminating to reflect on our fears, and level of risk and wonder, always wonder, Why? It seems from my earliest days, I learned in descent to be ultra cautious.

Why did I cry like a baby and freeze when my parents tried to have me climb down with them onto Cape Santa's overlook boulder? It was only a little rocky ledge that jutted out into the whirling Pacific sea?

Silly me, for even bringing these notes out here, but in moving aside like this, into the land of rambling reverie and questions of why, I discover light-bulbs of flashing insights. And it *is* funny in an odd way, when we catch the words that come to us to use in our storytelling.

The Lady of the Rock

Warmed and comforted by the brilliant, gathering radiation of the new day light, watching the sun rising ever higher in the sky, I was content to just sit and bask on that large slate-gray rock for a while. I rolled the sleeves of my T-shirt up to the top of my shoulders, pulled pants legs up above my knees, and tugged the collar down to better expose my throat and neck. It had been a long time since I had had the luxury of being bathed, warmed like this by the sun!

Never could I recall where it felt more natural.

Gentle breezes fanned and nudged from behind as the warm sun oriented and focused my gaze further deep on, into what was in front of me. I shifted onto my left hip until I felt a comfortable balance, finally resting at perfect still-point with my legs tucked alongside my right hip.

Secured by the safety of the rock, fed by the gentle breezes, warmed by radiation of the sun, I suddenly laughed out loud! My pose on that large rock reminded me of one of the two remaining sculptures my dad had fashioned over thirty years ago! We called her "The Lady on the Rock." Today she sits proudly as one of the focal points in our family room, symbolizing one of my few happier childhood times. In a rush of sweet melancholy, I recalled the happy joy my father had had when he was creating the Lady statue out of blocks of unpotentiated gray clay. Her rock, and the rock upon which I sat in the middle of the Blue Hills and Tye River, were the same slate color, boulder shape, and relative proportion to me. Dad had often said that he had seen me already all grown up—that the grown up Suzanne in his mind's eye had served as a model of the Lady for him.

> So here I was decades later, seated in repose and posed—
>> a life-sized reproduction of what he had created then—
>>> in form, she and me, born of far-sighted vision.

Overcome with the most exquisite, unspeakable awe, I replayed scenes of those days in full motion video with soundtrack, color, recalling happy feelings shared surrounding the creation, formation, and ultimate pride my father had when the sculpture was completed.

It was one of the very few father-daughter *heart* moments that we ever shared. And within that heart moment, those weeks from his visionary inception to final cast of the statue, he *caught* something he threw a long distance over time and across geography. While seated on the Tye River boulder, moving bolder to face Janus-like the past and future and oh, so totally in the present, I caught what he threw! And in my moment of surprise, my laughter sang out throughout the valley and beyond for all joy and comprehension of it all. The Lady on the Rock was one of our most profound, meaningful connections then and repeated long after his death, now. Synchronicity is not just another remarkable coincidence; it grabs us to the deepest core of being. At that dance point, we pirouette en pointe for all the understandings that rush forth, no less than the Sugarplum Fairy's dance of joy and mystery. After my morning hike up to the lower Falls, and exchanging energy with the wilderness back down along the mountainside, and gathering the vibrancy around me on the bridge, my cup was already running over that morning. To be lightning zapped, cracked, melted, dissolved, rooted, branched, and finally find myself grounded on the boulder mother rock in the exact pose of some long ago portrait-sculpture my father had conjured up in his creative mind, well, what else could I do, but laugh? The windows of the worlds had opened, and even at the most sweetest knowing, I knew that my dad and I, two timeless and essential souls, were connecting and communicating once again.

"Thank you, Daddy," I whispered to the river waters and butterflies surrounding me, "you are still one of the best teachers I have ever had!"

Immediately and simultaneously, upon that full musical scale of laughter recognition, the laughter surprise turned into a warm and comforting glow. I knew to my very core that my forever gratitude had been received, and had responded in like, in turn, by simply reflecting back to the source of that wonderful feeling the very glow I felt.

Heart to heart, soul to soul, mind to mind, I had connected with my essential father. And with that deep understanding I knew that this was not the physical man who had died shortly before his 43rd birthday and the roles he played, but rather a representation, a clustering of gathered, essential, integrated personalities. I would only discover the whole essence of the man on the days we connected as then, and only many years after my pain of our family's loss.

Similarities and paradoxical dichotomies, those meanings, understandings, lessons we shared? These had boomeranged, reverberated back and forward over time and place to meet, once again, at this place, on the rock and within my knowing place.

    As I resonated, vibrated, glowed, along those bypassed days,
        I received acknowledgment from
            all corners and extents of we-
ave,
                those past, present,
        future.
    Like a rallying cry, a call to home port
        consciousness converged again
    at that moment—
that dance point of still point when we combine
    integrate
        self song, each one's clear voice with
symphony,
        with synesthetic, combinations of pure
natural color of design,
        our threads, contributed,
            necessary and essential
those masterpieces and matter-flaws of the moment in the scheme of things
    the blink of an eye they say…
        well, dig deeply
            for our legacy of matter is but a
        blink of an I,
            and thrown down and up
            the winds of time,
        to spread over myriad places, to
    catch.

I was lucky, the Blue Hills called, and it was my time and place to catch a long pass from my father in hue-man terms. And just in case, to strengthen my holiday, all threads of the tapestry converged to butterfly language. From this point on, from personal to universal, I knew that I would catch their throw only when I became bolder and took those steps forward to visit their Island.

Haunting Memory

During Thanksgiving festivities when I was fifteen, and we were living in Death Valley, Mom and Dad really got into their celebration. We would make the stuffing and the side dishes (seasoned just so), iron and arrange the tablecloth, bring out the good dishes and family silverware. The big Thanksgiving meal was such a special family to-do that to this day, it is still the fondest holiday for me.

Anyway, on that particular Thanksgiving, Dad was in a touchy mood. His talking was difficult to follow as he waxed poetic, waned tearful, and roared rageful. Mom had already attempted suicide at least once and was already self-medicated. She was keeping a low profile that day. Both of them had enjoyed their whiskey and wine drinks during the fixing of the dinner. After the big turkey was placed in the oven, Mom went to take her afternoon nap. She had always slept at mid-day for as long as I could remember. Dad and I played a few games of chess to bide our time.

I grew itchy. Tired of chess and wanting to call my friends (or just withdraw to my room), I made the mistake of excusing myself from Dad's company. I did not want to learn again the special herbs and secret ingredients that went into the stuffing. I did not want to stick around and watch them get drunk and feel the tense vibes again.

    This type of talk was inexcusable.
        Dad blew up. He was beside himself.
            I tried to hide inside myself.
Then, during our cooling down period, he said that I must learn in my early years how to prepare "the big meal" just so, particularly the bird and stuffing. He emphasized and reiterated all of the do's and don'ts. For that, he said, was Mom's family specialty, the big meal; it was her Thanksgiving gift to us.

    Such a little thing to get angry about, I thought....
But his message was earnest and the following brief in passing.
        Because of his tone of voice, I paid special attention
            to his tone, timbre, and sincerity.

He shocked me then, when he said, "Learn what we can teach you now, because we won't be around much longer to help you out." Dad said his goal was to get me through High School, and so he did.

And then he died, and oh, how I cried, two weeks after my high school graduation. He never got to that special ceremony where I was awarded.

        There is something to be said for parents with far vision.

The Little Stone Path

The time had come. I felt like everything over these past two days, weeks and even a lifetime! had led up to this moment. No longer could I view life like some crazed TV surfer, hypnotized by the fragmented flashes of programming and sound bytes observed remotely, playing on without me on the big screen. My magic mountain area, with her butterfly trees, river, half moon bridge, and mother/ father rock, had called me here and invited me to play in my own role - my own script for this lifetime. Everything and everyone seemed to come together for this moment and all (yeah, right!) I had to do was follow the little stone path connecting this massive slate gray rock and walk onto shimmering iridescent
>   (purple
>   blue
>   green
>   gold
>   silver)

butterfly tree island to learn my destiny, and why I had been called.

Haunting Memory

In the movie *The Wizard of Oz*, Dorothy steps out from her black and white Kansas life and tornado-crashed house onto a fresh and magical, brilliant, Technicolor world—the Land of Oz. Munchkins serve as earth elementals, the "little people" who send her off on her archetypal journey. Each of the characters had a role to play and each was necessary to bring the whole story together in as many dimensions as the viewer wanted to explore. The story of the ruby slippers (tap three times and say, "there is no place like home", all the while living a dream within a dream of Home) is one of my favorites. And the familiarity of the people at home in Kansas to the characters she meets on her journey to Emerald City strikes quite a chord in me. The whole Wiz story is profoundly meaningful on many levels (I now see) and was a regular yearly family TV ritual (even before we had a color TV) when I was growing up. The show was usually aired in February's winter after my birthday. Predictably, the rainbow song cheered me up, because typically, I was down at that time with a bad cold!

Dances with Butterflies

     Ever encouraging me, a few of the more curious and courageous iridescent blues would venture over to my land, seeking me out while I continued to sit comforted and secure on that warming, nurturing boulder. Maybe they were attracted to my deep blue jacket and pale yellow T-shirt.

I smiled (to think) that they too might consider me a big mom butterfly
>
> who had mysteriously entered their
world.

They certainly were a curious and persistent lot!
>
> At times encircling as I followed one
>> and then another directly fly up to greet
> me face to face
>>> and then light alongside on one
>>> of the several smaller warming rocks to
>>> sparkle,

                          warm,

                                flex,

                                       and
                                  display their
                                  wings for a while.

Their patterns, their choices
>> —on which of the many
>> smaller rocks to pause—
>> revealed my own choices at that
>> moment.

     As they swirled around me, they outlined and occasionally lighted on the warm rocks rising slightly above the water to form a pathway.

The butterflies called (me) my attention to Nature's
nonrandom geometries;
        how the surrounding rocks architected a
perfect walkway
                between me perched on my
boulder
                and them dancing around on
their butterfly-tree island.

And how between us we formed one center
                of a shared universe together
        that radiated
                and linked stonestep
                walkways between us,
   the near and   the far shores,
                and the river fore and aft.

Artist Musings

Saying goodbye to the safe, solid mass of mother-father rock, I slid down the eastern side and stood facing directly into the sun. Straight ahead of me was the short connecting path of step-stone rocks in full shimmering aglow to butterfly tree island. Several of those (explorer) iridescent blues had already returned to home base to refresh and refuel.

Their invitation had been extended and it was time for me to accept. Feeling just like some sort of diplomatic emissary tasked no less than with the responsibility to learn all I could of their world and exchange what I could with them of ours, I crossed the bridge and finally stepped foot on the shore of butterfly-tree island.

An Aside

Somehow I already knew (when I stepped onto that Island) that my world would forever change. I was fully aware of my choice in the matter; this was not some "accidental" life changing experience that swept my roots out from under me and sent me swirling into outer space. My inner space had been prepared over a lifetime of all sorts of exceptional experiences, ranging from profoundly mystical to almost daily surprises of psi and synchronicity.

The past several years, especially, had been spent actively trying to make (create) some sense, some overarching pattern that would be meaningful and feel personally comfortable to me. Too, the past several months had been spent in intense email dialogs with my mother's sister, trying to reconcile my turbulent childhood to the person I am today, and to better understand the factors and personalities, my direct ancestral inheritance, that had shaped me in this life. The words that follow for the next segments, and the communications I received and acknowledged, will read and sound like science fiction and fantasy to those who have not shared these types of experiences. They will overlap with those who have had similar experiences, and read like a bad movie script to many! Nonetheless, this is what I stepped into and it is my story.

If this reads better as a story, and not as "the truth," then that is fine with me. At our essence, everything we communicate is a story, no more and no less, colored by our own perspectives, life experiences, cultural training and worldviews.

Going the Distance

Unlike being zapped by a lightning bolt that conducted through my body just minutes before, these first steps onto the land of the iridescent blues conveyed an embracing gentle warmth and muted golden glow within.

Yet it was an altogether different quality of warmth and glow from that of my Lady of the Rock experience. That boulder had embraced me, secured and grounded me to my elemental roots deep into the earth, into my own heritage. She offered safety and assurance that she would be forever there, rock solid, eroding and reshaping only gradually over the course of forever time, regardless of the powerful outside forces that constantly impinged and surrounded her. I was acutely and deeply aware of the various qualities of light, tone, hue, shading and tempo of each of my experiences over a lifetime, and how they enfolded together into this, my call to Life, exceptional human experience.

It was like this two day rest and relaxation had been exquisitely orchestrated with a symphonic virtuosity of some Maestro Conductor and yet, (no less) co-created, co-conducted (consciously or not) by me. Those first steps onto the foreign shore of butterfly island would be the result of all of those minute, shaping choices that I had made over a lifetime that had led ultimately (again) to this pivotal point.

Artist Musings

    Each encounter, each experience was an expression,
        and was altogether necessary and integral
            toward building and twining together
                the instrumental voice I carried
                    to harmonies and enfoldings
                      of the larger symphony of which I was a part.

    I fully understood at that moment that this was my choice.
        And, (profoundly) that it was also my responsibility.
        Otherwise, my voice would be forever lost amidst the cacophony of background surface noises--
those chaotic shrills   and basso dirges that stem from a meaningless life
        (of no perceived connecting theme, nor pulsar-rhythm, nor resonating harmony).

    Call me a romantic in rhapsody with Life, but I would rather dance with the rousing overtures and be at peace with the melodic largos, than deny my human birthright of full sensual awareness, and later regret having never really heard the music nor seen the colors of the world that constantly plays around, within, and through me.

Blue Hills Diary

PART IV: COMMUNION

Advancement

With small steady steps, I find myself on the brink of lost worlds. It is only with strength of will that I now advance. Unwavering, I move forward, now fortified and readied to forge whatever mountains and abysses lie ahead.

The Emissary

When I first stepped foot onto the foreign soil of butterfly-tree island, I was no less the explorer than was Neil Armstrong when he took his first tentative steps on the moon. It was a momentous occasion, a sort of summation of all of the relatively smaller steps that I had taken over the years to bring me directly to this place at this time. As an emissary to this new land, and a representative of my own, I was filled with the awesome responsibility to represent humankind in the clearest of lights that I could. I knew then that only by being a clear signal within myself could I hope to communicate, commune, with others who did not speak English, nor indeed any language that we would even remotely call "human."

Instead, I felt the need to communicate in a language that I had forgotten, but had had (daily) reminders and (nightly) retraining in it almost daily for as far back as I could remember (those ancient melodies). Of course, this new language immersion method was not always so obvious to me, the pupil. Rather, I must have absorbed enough over time to be fully present at that moment.

     Somehow I had passed the qualifying exam, applied for the position of communications specialist and was selected for this particular assignment. The *Who* (are you?) who had orchestrated with exquisite precision my first steps onto the (i)-land, my gathering awareness and dawning realization to my call has been called many names. Yet, by whatever name we address this Majesty that we have experienced in one way or another in our lives, we can agree on the universal numinous *quality* conferred and conveyed when we are in Its presence.

An Aside

    I fully realized that this was not an exploration to claim some piece of soil and its inhabitants for myself, my country, or my world. Rather, those first steps I took were wondrously symbolic to me and lent whole new levels of meaning to the worn, often meaningless phrases of

        gaining new ground
            and
                skipping the light fantastic.

    In one fell swoop I understood
            that I could have been anywhere
       at anytime and
           still received the same
           information.

       Paradoxically and exquisitely, I also understood
       that I was in the exact place and time,
           (just so aligned),
         that meaning connected
             the pieces of the puzzle
                of my life and
            thereby,
            and in that connection,
            I became fully conscious,
               fully aware,
                   of the role
               that I was to play.

Artist's Musings

Up to this point, these puzzle pieces had only been remote glimmers of color, hues, shadings, and seemingly random movements. Now, mere suggestions from those glimmer times gathered in shape to form an impressionistic picture as a whole. The movements, a fully orchestrated dance.

In the early times, there were no pieces to grasp from which I could anchor meaning on any form. These were felt as huge momentary blasts of indescribable illumination that would subsequently leave me speechless, spent, and longing for something.

Something that had no context, no moorings, no holds in which to even remotely relate to the events that had heretofore fashioned the painting,
>   the illusion
> of everyday life. Up to this point the impression of Life had been vague;
>> constructed by these glimmers
>>> and bursts of what can
>> only be called
>>> points of light and
>>> contrasting shadow.

And so, like the surprise and glee a child feels when her kiddie connect-a-dot drawing suddenly forms a recognizable picture, so too did my connect-a-dot painting, my calling to Life, suddenly come together out of the
> primordial

      stew of potential
           to take on a shape of its very
own.

      And that shape I recognized as me, my history, my evolution.

The seemingly random musical notes, like the picture dots, had been connected and what resulted at that moment was my melody, my leitmotif. Before, always haunting, just out of reach, and never quite resolved in its themes and variations, I suddenly heard, really *heard*, the
      signature theme
           that permeated (me) throughout
      my life
      and for the first time I recognized it and claimed it as my own.

Ancient Melody

     Ancient melodies pour forth again. These songs as ancient as the blue hills I now walk upon. I know not whether I am seeing the distant past or the coming future.
     I ask the perennial questions—
          Why I am here to be?
               What of this question of soul?
     Answers are primal, mythical to some—rational debate for others.
     Yet, now I feel these answers as songs sung deeply,
          creations imprinted some way when time no longer mattered,
               to unfold and resurrect now in my remembering place.

     I stand on the hillside with many of my clan surrounding.
     We await the visitors who arrive
         in vehicles different than the twentieth century cars
              where physical bodies are not necessary to gain access
                  or be seen.
     The lights of the night sky are closer that evening,
                  it is a late summer's eve
            when the rosy-indigo twilight is settling
               to ground, shading us
               prematurely, encircling us,
               protecting us
                  from whatever is to come for Earth.

We are at one location of many communication
ports—
    the wheeled hubs, interconnecting
spokes within wheels—
        points forming ley meridians of
alternating
            electric and magnetic
energy
                similar to those
            marked within our own
            bodies.
            (We had forgotten.)

The people gather; we now become our true,
soul selves
    —the energy wheels of humankind—
    no longer needing the
reminders of the ritual
        posed by building
Medicine Wheels
            or Fairy Rings
            discovered wherever in
            surprises.

We pay tribute and listen well, the sounds of
the twilight suddenly hush
    as the evening sky overhead turns and
revolves,
        the points of light shifting
overnight in one second
            in one moment of truth,
        remembrance.
        But we are not afraid
            for we know
        and follow this, our calling.
                It is Time.

The Language of Butterfly

Upon my first steps onto butterfly-tree island, realizations flashed quickly into being, at once both recognized and written in indelible ink. I understood at that moment that my task when I returned home was to recapture in writing the full experience of the Blue Hills and to convey as best I could in words this precious Knowledge.

Stepping forward, full face into the brilliant warm sun, I followed the short narrow pebble stone path that led me directly into the shimmering land of butterfly. No longer a distant impressionist's painting upon which I could gaze at my leisure from afar, I now walked directly into that canvas and became fully essential, integral, to that vibrant work of art that had called me.

After only a few steps, I stopped to pause between the two huge honeysuckle bushes. They stood on either side of me, gently brushing my arms and hips with their heavy summer-laden tangled branches, and dripped their golden yellow blossoms into my face. I stood mesmerized, as scores of iridescent blues and monarch yellows and pristine whites swirled and glittered all around me in the sunshine. Only my eyes moved as I watched first one and then another, and then a duo, dance and weave in and out of my view. So close, they were, that I could feel their breezy flutter and hear their heartbeat wings strumming the air.

Fully at peace and fully in the timeless moment, I suddenly realized that they had captured me into their own butterfly net! Our roles and our worlds had been reversed. Now they were the scientists observing and gathering field data about me and my habits. And there I was, a most unlikely specimen who had been singled out, baited by their beauty and flushed into their net.

I smiled upon that realization and glow-beamed a signal of grateful warmth out to them. Remarkably, in tandem, several butterflies paused in their swirling activity. Instead of continuing to circle around, each lighted upon a nearby flower or honeysuckle branch and stopped to rest, warm, and flex its wings. Their sudden halt in activity gave me a bit of a giggle. The butterflies were playing like children. Each scrambled to find a seat in a game of musical chairs. Yet instead of music being stopped to signal a change in the ongoing activity, somehow my warm glow of gratitude projected out to them had been received. They rested expectantly, warming and flexing their blue wings, each claiming a seat positioning at different intervals and distances from me. Remarkably, they were ready to communicate, acknowledging my glow-beam with a glow back in response! I was simply stunned! And then amazed, for in the language of butterfly, they had received my glow communication and they had acknowledged and reciprocated in like.

How did I know this? I just *knew*. This too was a game. In first contact, we just dropped the boundaries between us and just got into the play of it all.

Glow to warm glow, we continued to build and expand the link that was being fashioned between us. That link, that language, was uniquely butterfly. As an emissary to their land, I needed to learn their language, and live fully immersed within their culture to better understand their message. Theirs is a soft and gentle glow; subtle with flickering flashes comprised of powerful, fleeting bits of instantaneous knowledge about the cycles of life and death—of painful, wrenching transition and glorious transformation. Because their life cycle is brief, their time consciousness is wholly different from human.

>
> To understand the language of the butterfly,
> the human communicator must slow
> way down, to
> step
> down
> time
> in such a way as to Stop!
> human time
> in a series of
> freeze frames.

For this was our dance—to gather and then connect
moments to anchor moment,
for next moment to moment,
and so on, soon—
in the world of
butterflies.

Too, their world is local, spanning only the distances necessary to
cocoon,
drop,
crawl,
and fly
in short bursts during the warm
shines of day,

and to rest safely in the silences of the dark night.

From the perspective of human,
> they are restricted to short times and small spaces,
>> but are we any less in our own lives?

Those iridescent blues gifted me with a most profound and powerful message that day. The continuation of this diary as a series of moment to moment experiences was born from their very invitation,
> their persistence,
> their net,
>> their wisdom,
>>> and their miracle.

An Aside

Butterflies helped me remember, in the most literal sense of the word. They reminded me that each moment has a greater depth, an essential quality to share that is often discounted, skimmed over, rationalized, or called "forgotten" in our human way of the world.

They taught me that every moment is heavily pregnant with meaning, and to enter their world and the worlds outside of our limited scope, all we need do is to be receptive - enter into that quality (an essentially different time) and speak the language of that (seemingly foreign) world. I had forgotten how many times I had done this over my (now) lifetime, to really feel the different sensitive qualities, to connect and communicate at different levels being to being to Being.

But the butterflies did not let me forget this time, because it was my time to remember. Magic mountain had called me. She had magnetized me to her place. I finally got the message to return. And, in my returning, I recalled my song as being one of communicator—a translator and interloper between the worlds, as my mother taught me. I share these messages with you today in real time, as they unfold from within me.

One backward, forward, and inside-out dance that was originally infused to unfold over the years from those two magnificent September days and nights in the Blue Hills.

Unfurl

*Each being called a
name.*

*Each name called a thing
including human beings who,
or the mountain it, or the stars
they,
we all--
be-ing beings who share
this Earth called It to
some and Her to many
now
understanding the
vibrations
of quality differentials
across time zones
and cycles
those Universal essential
qualities
that make the world go around.*

*The birds and the bees, the butterflies they
are also who's, as are the flowers and
sand and rocks and trees.*

*While Mother Earth conjuncts and communes
with Father Sky
(and Moon daughter's speaks her
monthly words)
their silent coupling joins in
rhythm to
our own inner
communication.*

The very magi stars, other constellations, they speak to us,
> *to our waters for dolphins and whales and frogs and fishes,*
> *and terrestrial habitats for humans beings and all creatures*
> *two by two, manifold by many folding (even the extinct ones)*
>> *(considered sentient or not).*

>> *All Universal*
>>> *One Song*
> *across species, respected, respective here and now, there and then.*

> *Listen well!*
Hear too our Universal sound bytes, these communions
>> *between our glorious variety of specie qualities and times.*

The Butterfly Dance

How long did we communicate like this, bouncing glow-beams back and forth? I really cannot say, even to this day. As I gradually entered the time and the world of butterfly, such questions had no meaning. We had created and blended our own time, based solely on the quality of glow we shared between us.

We expanded the web and grew our connection into ever faster cycles of pulsing glimmers, until all was one continuous channel, a continuous stream of light. In contrast to the back and forth that we humans use to universally punctuate and construct our own sense of time, we had fashioned a sort of fiber-optic link of our own. This link, comprised solely on a steady stream of mutual consciousness, is best translated as a specific *quality* of light that we shared.

Amazingly, that bandwidth, that channel of streaming light, was propelled by intent (magnetic to one, electric from one) energy. It *flowed both ways simultaneously* and information was just there with no differentiation as to the "who" who sent or acknowledged, or the sequencing of "whens."

Information, Knowledge between us just was.

An Aside

Something quite magical happened to me that morning. At first blush, it all started with being zapped on that mountain path, when I realized why I had been called there and then. Magical is as good a word as any to convey the "now you see it, now you don't" feeling between ecstasy and afterglow.

One feeling similar to when a magician makes a rabbit disappear by waving a scarf in front of it, and Voila! No more rabbit.

First there is
    and then there isn't,
        and we either enjoy the wonder
of it all
        or more likely,
           we begin to
        question *how* did he do it?
        What happened in that in-between stage?

That butterfly communication was a strange one though. Instead of something there and then just magically disappearing, this was more of a
    "now you don't see it,
        now you do"
           a reversed sort of thing.

Haunting Memory

After our move to Friday Creek, Lee and a couple of my closest friends from Anacortes came for a visit and to spend the night. It was my birthday. Birthdays were honored in our home by a special dinner, a special homemade cake and some form of acknowledgment that another year had passed.

My girlfriends thought the bungalow house real cool, a lot of fun,
> because at the solid oak bar with built in barstools
>> we could ride round and round
> 'til vertigo dizzy
>> clockwise and
> counter-clockwise
>> with just a push off of one foot or the other.
>> (If our legs were long enough for a good spin).

Anyway, after the feasting followed by cake and ice cream, Dad showed us his magic act. You know, the simple one? The one where a coin disappears and suddenly appears from behind one of our ears? Or, when we discover to our glee that it reappears in the magician's other hand?

Well, that was a hit, he had us all oohing and aahing, warmed up for the special show. The highlight of the getting-to-be-late night was when we were all in a circle, sitting comfortably on the floor, Dad too. Mom was nearby, keeping track of the goings on whilst she surreptitiously cleaned up from our banquet of deep fried shrimp, French fries and cake dinner.

>(Oh, no worry over the fat and cholesterol then!)

My sister was, as usual, somewhere. I don't recall whether she joined us girls or not. Probably not. I was pretty impatient with her in our growing-up days, and my friends were my friends. Hers? Well, she had none her own age and took a yen to the old, kind couple who lived across the bridge on the other side of Friday Creek. They lived hidden deep in the depths of the woods, a bit of a mystery as I remember now— remembering their familial warmth and reclusive ways. But that is written in another book, a teen mystery story to tell someday, with clues still locked in the nooks and crannies of my memory and the old bungalow home.

For the big act, my father had us sit just so, as he did, on the floor in a circle, and then placed his Zippo lighter in the center between us all. The trick was to make the lighter move by just thinking that it *had already* moved, and concentrate...

>Oh! Concentrate!
>>on that lighter moving in one direction or another
>>>(the direction being voted by us first).
>>And Wow! in the middle of the dark candlelit room,
>>>where the *Monkey's Paw*

story had just been told,
we girls saw the lighter shimmer and then skim
the surface of the
hardwood floor,
inching its way, in some way, toward someone.
An early lesson in mind-
over-matter, not forgotten.

Unfurl

Even the magician was surprised.
> *There was another Magic at work.*

I wondered about the before and after and the in-between
> *of that zap-stream of Light that had me anchored*
>> *deep into the core of magic mountain and at the same time*
>>> *beamed me straight out into the cosmos.*

> *No missing time. Time stood still.*
> *No missing information,*
> *Knowledge was infused.*

That this Knowledge is still with me and continues to unfold,
> *as I write these words, is a source of precious, magical wonder to me.*

For those looking for the exact moment of that pivotal experience,
> *that transformative moment of in-between,*
>> *it was around 9.20 that morning*
> *EDT*
> *And exactly a lifetime...*

But when I stretch that time
>> *and move moment to moment, moment to moment*
>>> *(as the butterflies had taught me)*
>>>> *I realize*
>>> *that there were many, many magical moments*

before and
after
that constellated, gathered together in that single mystical experience.
The befores, no longer befores; and the afters, no longer afters.
Rather, only One
extraordinary continuous moment
that somehow found its alpha and omega in the in-between.

A still point of peace that manifested,
be-came to life, alive and living,
through me.
Like the wheel snake, where the alpha head circles around to meet the omega tail and form a continuous feeding hoop, time no longer is seen as a straight arrow line of past, present, future. Yet we can still recognize that symbol as a snake swallowing its tail.

We ask: What came first, the chicken or the egg?
I don't know, there are arguments for each side
(as if chicks and eggs have sides).
But when we no longer see sides, and begin to see them only as convenient constructs useful to communicate amongst ourselves,
we once again return to our wholeness and our very holiness.

An Aside

I have always as a natural preference to view the whole as contiguous connecting patterns, then segment and slice that whole into its contributing parts to better communicate. On the other hand, some people prefer to build patterns creating the whole out of its representative parts.

Both "types" of mind are essential and necessary to the discovery of that magical moment, that flash point of catalytic insight and meaning. Simultaneously building up and breaking down to where we find our peace, our still point where heaven and earth meet within ourselves. It is simply miraculous and enchanting! And wholly contained within us.

In the blink of an eye, we are both mother and child fully present at our own quickening and the world is forever transformed.

Presto! Changeo! The "who" who we were before is not the "who" we are after.

We have formed *yet another*
bridge between worlds
where self meets Self, reconnects and
remembers.

Connected to these many worlds within, we connect with those many worlds without—from the personal to the mundane to the cosmic. At that moment of what can only be called *infused Knowing,* we are at once both the center of the Universe and all extensions and possibilities. The symbol of the bridge is as good as any to mark here to there and back again. Yet, at that point of the in-between, we are free to move in other dimensions, forward and back, up and down, side to side

                        (forward, backward, inside out).

      We discover our personal portals that connect us to infinite worlds. And, having forged a secure foundation of our own within and between here to there, we are reassured that when we venture out to commune with other worlds

and walk other bridges
           (high and low)
    we will once again return,
    safely and intact, to familiar Home territory.

Harmonic Note

Timeless Knowledge; stories journaled in symbol and meaning for as far back as humankind can recall. Stories of exploration chronicled in cave dwellings and on stony petroglyphs, within sacred temple architectures, in the geometry of massive stones, where modern rituals have lost their meaning.

Captured in perennial literature, philosophies, human masterpieces of art, music, and dance.

The Blue Hills

The sun continued to warm and nurture me as I stood amidst those sweet scented honeysuckle trees, communing with those shimmering blue butterflies. By mid-morning, the day was fast approaching another record high to the mid-90s. The oppressive heat and humidity were quite unusual for this mountain climate that third week of September. Once again I was glad that I had taken an early morning route.

On occasion, I could hear a car making its way up the mountain slope to join the range along the exposed backbone of the Blue Ridge Parkway. The Blue Ridge route spans from southern Virginia and northern North Carolina, connecting the Shenandoahs of the north to the Great Smoky Mountains of the south. Collectively this range, called the Appalachian Mountains, spans the whole length of the eastern mountain divide of the continental United States. It was incredible for me to realize that I had hiked on various segments of that mountain range from Maine to Georgia over the past thirty years. And that here I was again, just a mile or so from another looming peak, where in some way my footsteps had connected time and returned once again to this particular place.

The earth weathered; her hills had grown ancient. They were formed and shaped by nature's elements over vast seasons out of time. Millions of individual footsteps had trekked the Appalachian Trail between here and there. By the time I visited the island and communed with the butterflies, my footsteps on her mountain slopes already rested, embedded, and had been imprinted with countless others, including my former steps upon that very path where I had walked years and eons before.

Artist Musings

Oh, the butterfly color! Here, another encounter with that particular shade of deep shimmery blue-violet again! I just can't escape it and thus have made my choice to embrace it, learn from it. So while I was communing with my otherworldly guides, wearing their guise in butterfly wings, I asked "Why?"

Amazing what answers we receive when we just ask a simple straightforward question like "Why?" In a heartbeat, all of the times and places where I had vibrated to that particular shade, that particular nanometer of measured wavelength of iridescent blue, flashed onto my own inner silver screen and connected the dots. What a starry constellation of flashbacks! Grounded human in golden yellow-orange, my spiritual self is ported via silvery blue-violet. During those times over my lifetime, when I travel to realms outside of my physical self, that particular shade of iridescent blue heralds these shifts.

You know that color? (Do you know "Blue Star"?) That blue-green-violet shade of an alexandrite gemstone or perhaps a tanzanite that can only be seen for what it is worth when the light shifts prisms of colors within? It is that degree, that particular color of shading, which scintillates just beyond and beneath the surface. I have often caught this will o' wisp of color moving in and out of my everyday sensory vision. Sometimes it manifests in the guise of a butterfly wing, or as a bird's feather, a particular flower, perhaps a gemstone gift—and once it fell from heaven to earth as a blue-green fireball star before my very eyes.

It is at those times that I know I have been blessed. Something greater than me is at work. Yes! Yet I also know that I am somehow essential, necessary to *Its* conveyance from meaningless random nothings into meaningful patterned somethings. Vision is nothing until it is a creation in form.

In one clear light-beam with the butterflies, I recalled all of the times when this particular shade of blue had come into my life. I had learned that this color heralds special "pay attention" times—more to follow. While I stood transfixed in the sun on the island that day, the assembled butterflies swarmed and once again took flight around me. They circled around me once again and then, amazingly, that glow between us began to stretch, as the butterflies took flight higher up and farther out. As the glow between us expanded, I too could feel myself expanding, rising, above the rocky island.

Up, up, I floated, above the lush verdant canopy of summer-laden trees draping over the Tye River. Gliding, floating on gentle wafts of sunlit air, blue butterfly glow carried me downstream, to greet the rising sun. I return once again, back in time.

Haunting Melody

We had little time, my father said. Life at the Navy base on the desert's edge of Death Valley and having to deal with Mom's growing distancing from the world had tired us all out. But the solution Dad suggested seemed bizarre to this fifteen-year-old girl. The cure seemed worse than the malady. He suggested that we withdraw from society altogether.

The plan was to find a hidden spot in the Ozark (the Oz and the Ark) Mountains, build our own house in the trees, live on bags of grains, and take a library of books to last us for years to come. Almost immediately, Mom agreed with Dad's plan to withdraw from the world at large and for the four of us learn to survive in the wild. The only thing that even came close in my imagination was those visions of Tarzan of the Jungle. My parents wanted a safe haven where we would live with the animals as human animals. The daily routine would be to build a tree house, forage food and stave off interlopers. We would be picking berries and stripping bark from trees, fishing for trout or perhaps catching a possum in a trap for dinner. The grains in the bags would be mixed with water, or milk from our own cow, and we would be feasting on flour mush and stale pancakes every day. Yummy!

A most unappetizing thought.

The family talked on at length about this plan for several months. It was amazing to see Mom and Dad so animated and yes, even excited, rejuvenated, about it all. They had even worked the math details and accountancy at length, working well into the nights, over weekends, only pausing to ask me questions off and on to fill the order.

To say it mildly, I was not enthused. I tried to be. I even got books out of the town library about the old South and mountain-life in the 1960s. My parents would teach me, they said; no formal schooling was necessary. All I could see was boredom ahead.

Although the Ozarks weren't the Blue Hills, the concept of mountain living, with its sanctuary and retreat from life's stresses, was born in those days.

Haunting Melody

The police came to get me one night when I was folk dancing at the community clubhouse in Death Valley. Folk dancing was a regular Thursday evening activity for me. It was an out-of-the-house event with a much more stable adult crowd who welcomed us kids to join them. Oh, how much I enjoyed those days of international dancing in my early teen years! When the police arrived, they asked some of the older, wise men where I was.

To my absolute horror, they began walking toward me (smiling, friendly, encouraging). I already *knew* somehow, in some way, that they had come (in full uniform) for me, but hoped against hope that it was not true.

(A kind of a gut wrenching knowing it was—you know what I mean).

Anyway, they located me and gently walked me off the dance floor. They wanted to talk about my folks and to give me a ride home.

Mom was in the hospital, with an overdose of pills that time,
                   and Dad was by her side at the hospital.
    She was touch and go.
 Strange, all seemed pretty "normal" when I left the house earlier that evening.
 Perhaps she was just putting on a good act. Who knew? I sure didn't. But the police? Now, this was serious business. They even asked me whether my

father had ever hurt my mother. They asked whether
my parents had even argued that day.
> No way, I said, not even a peep of anger
between them, ever, never, even.
>> The truth, I said, was that
>>> they never ever even
>> argued—
> It was their badge of honor, no fighting
between them,
>>> at least of the vocal or
>> physical kind.
>> The house usually was quiet as
> a tomb
>>> except for the TV talking
>> or recorded music singing
>>> —and the occasional
>> schmaltz of a lost (soul) violin.

(My sister has a different story of those days
and the later days that came and went, but it seems
that I was never at home during those times when our
parents staged an all out war of words and some
flinging of arms.
> No marks that I could see—perhaps
they were well hidden.)

The police, satisfied with my version of our family's
usually placid environment, drove me home and called
Dad.
> Dad tried to be calm and yet was beside
himself at the same time.
> He said that all Mom could do was sleep now
and mend.
>> I heard his weeping frustration
>> and the very pain of hurt
>>> leaking through his voice.
>>> I felt his

enormous fear and deep
love for Mom.
He was at an absolute loss; her scream
for help so drastic.
The family boat had been
rocked, and from then on
after her public
demonstration of supreme pain
(touching both
ways to four ways)
the spirals
spiraled down for
us all
to a place where we were
left, gasping for fresh air.
Our family's door had been
tightly shut,
with the glue of family
life, secrets shared—
a life now shattered, dispersed, broken—
made public on record for all to see
our silent
seal of what had been
once
securely
locked
within.

Nowhere to go, nowhere to hide, Mom compensated and tried to pay penance for her public demonstration of pain. From there on out, she played her role as the sick one; reclusive for the rest of her short miserable life. In the meantime, Dad moved up to protect her and his girls in any way he could. He became the sole wage earner, moving out into the world at large, demanding a fair play in a world that demanded a college degree as tithe. That degree, he did not have. The world was not interested in others.

     In life's game of chess, I too shifted to become the parent of my parents, and left my little sister more or less to fend for herself. As her physical disabilities became more apparent—and ignored—she was often left out in her preteen years
     except for her expression of love for the Sunday evening TV show *Lassie*
and we all in unison lifted a > right paw of friendship to that faithful and courageous collie dog.

Unfurl

Revisiting those childhood days still makes me sad and anxious.
This is not a novel unfurl, many families have had their pains to overcome,
but it is *such a test of replaying those emotional climates—*
*real again in order
to write these words
of how I was
shaped by my early
years—*
*whether
these words will
ever
make a formal
story or not,
(or read like one long run-on sentence).*

*These haunting types of entries are the most difficult,
they rub my soul and heart raw.
And in that rawness,
I feel again
the depths of the very great abyss.*

Haunting Memory

Home life and school life did not mix. At home I was learning parental responsibility for my parents and at school I tried to excel in my studies to make them proud of me. I was a pleaser. At home, I learned to keep my head low and do my chores. Don't rock the boat, I learned, don't start a sudden uproar. At school, it was important to be popular (which meant being extroverted, joining a variety of clubs and activities) and escaping when I could to the proffered sanctuaries of my friends and their homes. This pattern of separating home life from school life was already well entrenched by the ninth grade.

After moving to two houses over three years on the navy base in the middle Death Valley, Mom began her swan song in earnest. She was losing ground and sinking fast.

After her massive overdose of prescription pills, it seemed that nothing could soothe her. Electrical shock treatments (ECS) over the years to come would prove no exception. Lord knows, we all tried and she tried most of all. But drinking was her substitute when the surrounding emotional climate got rough. Her sensitivity to the subtle currents of discontent surrounding our family at home would continue to get the best of her. And I now suspect, in retrospect, that she was also very much attuned, in some intangible way, to what was going on outside of our immediate home base—into the realms of those unspoken strategies which served the overall mission of the navy base we lived on in those days.

So on July 4th weekend 1967
      (three years exactly to the day plus one day
           when Dad would die),
we gathered our things into the car and were on the road again.

An absolute surprise to me, the shocking suddenness of it all! I didn't even have time to say goodbye to my school friends that summer, but the folk dancers got hugs all around.

Behind the scenes, Dad had secretly planned a cross-country trip for us—
      one family trip of no return—
        that began from the
southwest Mojave Desert,
      driving old Route 66,
      leading into more fiery hell.
      The joys of Route 99 left far behind
      in this young girl's mind
at the soul banks of Friday Creek.

There would be no time for touring on this trip, or visiting any Elks lodges along the way. It was a straight shot—a whirlwind trip. Our original destination was Little Rock, Arkansas, to find a new home, get some financial footing with the help of Dad's Dad.

(That move lasted only four days before we were told to move on.)

We stayed at a colonial white-house-with-pillars motel and called it home, while all the while Dad and his dad negotiated their options. Mom, in the meantime, was at the point of drinking shaving lotion. Granddad would have none of that nonsense in *his* town around his second wife. So we packed up our clothes, loaded our bags
    and were on the road again.

        This time our nomadic destination was Washington, DC
                (somewhere around
            there)
            anywhere where Dad's
        personnel work
                and government
            experience
might help land him a job.

Sis and I, we got to stay in Pitt County, NC with Dad's Mom for a few weeks while our parents drove on, north to DC, to locate our new home,
        a chance of income for Dad
                and to soothe Mom's most
        desperate pleas for help.

The drive that summer of '67 was over a rough, rough road. My jobs were to dole out two-finger whiskeys with one ice cube each from the back seat of the car upon request from either Mom or Dad, watch Mom like a hawk during the times Dad had to go somewhere, and try to keep my little sister amused during the insanity of it all. These were full time jobs. Books became increasingly vital to my sanity.

Jeane Dixon's *A Gift of Prophecy*, I recall, was a hit that summer.
> It felt familiar too,
>> the modes of psychic she was writing about.
>>> I already had had impressions and visions
>>>> for as long as I could remember.

An Aside

There have been too many goodbyes in my life. The shields outside and the armor inside are now forged strongly against that kind of pain. Death takes my friends and family, even a family pet, and I am devastated once again. How does one overcome the perpetual hurt of loss?

It is easier to cry when a cat or dog, or even a roadside animal, is hurt or sick or dies than a fellow human being these days. Why? Maybe I do not want to write about that final gate. That would be the simple answer. Yet my mind still reasons in the magical world of the child at times. For those times, beginning in my earliest years, I wondered: Was it possible that somehow, in some way, I may have inadvertently *caused* a death of someone I so deeply love?

It is that pain, nested within this story of wonder, I share with you. No wonder transcendence fills the minds of us who worry with the weight of "*Alas*" on our shoulders.

Suzanne V. Brown, Ph.D.

Haunting Memory

By 1967, the writing had been written on the subway wall, our sometimes tenement hall. While Simon and Garfunkel sang of their old friend "Darkness," Mom continued her silent scream of desperation, seeking soothes for help. Dad was beside himself, for he did not know what to do to help her. They danced a dramatic tango back and forth, full of promises; succumbing to broken links and renovating romantic reconciliation, while our family of four learned to dance the quadrille.

After our move to Arlington, Virginia, the job that was to be there for Dad, wasn't. I learned then that a college education was essential. I saw what happened to a genius man who traveled to the beat of his own drum and was turned down time and time again for the lack of that piece of ruled sheepskin. It took Dad seven months to land his dream job, but he got it when he had nothing left to lose. It was perfect for him! A job that he had been wanting for a long time: personnel director of a hospital. His dream was to return to medicine in his off-hours, to putter around the labs and learn some of the newer technologies that had developed since his days in Anacortes. Mom and we girls were thrilled for him! Moreover, we could begin to rent furniture again, after seven months of having tables set on orange crates and sleeping on floor pallets. We had made an exception, however, with a rented TV that kept us entertained during those in-between times.

For me, entertainment was high school, of course. My sophomore year began that autumn and kept me entertained, and entertaining. I was a novelty to my new friends—a long-haired blonde, a California girl, who had been transplanted into the old South and fashionable East. Talk about culture shock! Those were the days when California dreaming, surfer songs and "love-ins" began crossing the United States from West to East. During this backward motion, when social forces moved retrograde against Earth's turning of time and collided in the hurricane winds of fiery civil unrest that peaked that summer in 1967, I learned the human meaning of west meets east. To bridge backward to our roots, is to foster forward growth for our branches.

And so it goes—

backward,

forward, and inside out.

No matter how tough things were financially, we always had food in the pantry. No matter what fate brought our way, even in our leanest days at Friday Creek, Dad promised us that we would never go hungry, and we never did.

Yet Mom continued her fall downstream. Caught in a current of no return, she lost all peace of mind, for her soul had been filled by those murky, self-destructive demons of her own creation. Regardless of any happy news shared by us, it was transitory—family joys were mere ripples against the gathering tides that were sweeping her out to sea. Her gentle nature had succumbed. Her creative, childlike spirit had been displaced. Beyond any call for help, she had forgotten how to walk like an Indian in gentle toe-heel steps amongst ever-changing, new terrain. Instead, her inner anguish began to pound heavily upon the earth to be heard by all of us. She extracted pounds of flesh from each of us for supposed past payments due.

For reasons I still try to understand, she demonstrated her pain only when I was present. Via a variety of suicide attempts, these acts of desperation would be staged only when she and I were alone in the house.

Oh dear Mother, why me? What in the world, or out of it, were you trying to tell me in those days? What had I missed?

My little sister would be outside playing, still at school, or in her room. Dad, predictably, would be at work at the hospital. More often than not, Mom attempted suicide in the late afternoons while I was doing my homework or coming home after being out with friends. There she would be, exhibiting all sorts of creative self-destruction.

      She was hopeless, in the true sense of that word
          and I was helpless to help.

            Her gathering drunk, crying, never raging—
              sticking her head in the gas oven,
              or popping extra bottles of prescription pills
            (each of her doctors did not know of the others),
              or on one fine spring day,

                 I came home to find her
      slicing (timing) through her wrists with the
carving knife.

      I was Mom's caretaker. The pills were hidden in the basement, near the very place where we took turns practicing the violin. She would beg me for just one pill more. In the meantime, taxi drivers would deliver whiskey or beer or wine whenever she had a dollar or two to spare. These drivers got her well on her way, early in the day, way before I returned from school.

      But sticking her head in the gas oven made me so very angry
              it was staged to get my attention
              when I was faced backward, away from
the kitchen,

                            attempting to learn a new
                chess situation.

    And the worst
            was her slicing through the meaty veins
of her wrists
               till they oozed rich red blood,
      why?
Why, did she do it?

            Why, the *when* did she choose to do it?
              Why that day when I was
        bringing a friend to visit after school?
                  I was seventeen, with a
                    friend waiting at the door,
                 when Mom

                decided to carve
                her wrists into
                mincemeat.
Perhaps I had disobeyed?
      The Rule of the house was that it was off limits to friends
             without prior permission from
      Dad.
             (We kept our family secrets to
      ourselves.)

So, while Mom was slicing into her wrists, and before they spewed, I ran back to the front door to tell my girlfriend a little white lie—Mom was sick and I had to take care of her. There would be no talking about boys or homework studies for us that afternoon. My friend left quickly, taking note of my suddenly cool, collected, responsible face. My school friend got the hint, with little explanation, bless her heart!

In growing anguish, I shut and locked the door, and quickly switched gears back to home territory. There was family business to attend to. Racing back to the kitchen, Mom and I tussled over the whiskey bottle. She lost. I applied a tourniquet with a dishtowel to stop the bleeding and patched Mom's wrists. I had learned first aid early on from both of my parents. Then I poured what was left of the cheap bourbon, with its sour butterscotch odor, down the sink. Mom was shaking and pleading for just one more drop. I had to stand firm; I had to say no. I had been instructed.

Then I called Dad at work. He was at his new job with the hospital and could not come home early that day.

He had done that too many times before,
        riding in on his white horse
           in the guise of a desert-
        sand colored Rambler American.
That day, Mom's demonstration was just one more motion
        —one more expressive emotion—
of desperation that proved too much for us.

I am not sure if my sister ever knew of that turning point day when Mom and I danced once again the ballet of life and death, reenacting our roles of martyr and savior.
    (The weight of Alas rests heavy on our shoulders.)
Dad said that I had handled the situation well. He praised me for my quick thinking in an emergency.
    (Keep it in the family.)
A new pattern of dynamics was etched clearly in my mind from that day forward. From then on out, after that turning point,
    I became the full caretaker of my mother
        and soothsayer to my father,
           for he was at a loss
                and could take no more.

Ancient Melody

       Death is but a doorway
            I have walked through many
times before.
       Those times of reverie
            how to communicate the ease,
the simplicity?
       Hands reach out to welcome me.

Butterfly Transforms

I followed the butterflies as they rode
       along the warming updrafts of Tye River
breezes.

They were
            darting in and out,
                  playfully crossing
            back and forth and
                always
            just a little bit in
            front of me.

They wove
            a web by their crossing,
              and crisscrossing,
                weaving in a
            bubble of time-space
            glow.
            (They invited me to follow
their lead.)

I felt safe and protected within our fashioned
bubble of light
    knowing that my physical self
        was still happily standing on the
island path
            while my "flights of
fantasy"
                were projecting
        back in time and
downstream
            to one
of the most magnificent encounters with
iridescent blue
I have ever had in my life.

    This dance too, would be one
        of those major turning points of
my life.
    And those journeys had taken place
        within the space—
            a mere fraction of a mile
away
            from where my
        body remained still,
standing mute— in a place
called *No Time*.

Critical Mass

I absorb the nature of earth and heaven surrounding me and recognize its reckoning of my day soon to end. The build-up of tensions even of the most divine kind cannot be ignored and my choice is to survive. Once again I bid farewell and withdraw from a most precious place in order to escape the intensity that would otherwise scatter me widely, unnamed and untamed. I am not discouraged.

It was time to return back to the little homey motel and rest up, integrate my morning's experiences. To be zapped on the mountainside and commune with the butterflies was more than one day's, a lifetime's, reckoning. I left butterfly-tree island the same way I had come, backwards now. Turning tiny pivots on each of the stones and toe-hugging once more, I beamed my goodbyes out to Mother-Father rock. The iridescent blues followed me out, circling wider and wider, as I traced my line of return back to solid ground.

I had requested solitude on the mountain and was grateful that my request had been granted. No other humans had crossed my path that morning. No other cars had turned into the parking lot of Crabtree Falls during those early hours.

It was only when I stepped back onto the pavement to return to my car that another car pulled up. The timing was exquisite! And even more so was my delight when the young couple who had emerged from their car told me that they had missed the sudden left < turn into the parking area. Because of this, they had arrived at least fifteen minutes later than they expected.

> (It is all in the timing, and we are not the timekeepers.)

They told me that they had already gone to the top of the ridge, where the meadows were, and had to cycle back in order to hunt for the missing entrance they had missed when driving up the hill.

Amazing when we are in tune with, in dance with, the Universal song. I had asked for solitude and received it. The young couple's arrival was right on time for me, and I suspect, for them. I wonder if that timing meant anything to them? For me, it was proof that enchantment was fully present. The Blue Hills had called me and I had answered their call. I had returned to my sacred place. Old cycles within new cycles had connected and fused within me. And there was no telling, then, about how far ranging the fusion of broken links into a whole design would take me.

Nor would I ever know to what extent my own reconnection, transformation, in the form of zaps and glows, sudden realizations and insights, would ripple across time and space to mend the wounds of others and the Divine Creation we all are.

Back in the World

After that morning of the second day, I fairly flew down the twisty road that had, only hours earlier, led me up to Crabtree Falls. On the way back, I pulled a right > turn into the campgrounds for a moment to revisit the medicine wheel that we girls had built eleven years before, but the owners had changed. They had gated off their property from casual sightseers (or from any seers for that matter).

Wanting to keep my peace of mind and determination to be solo on this journey, I backed out of their drive and continued down the mountain—leaving the blue hill that housed the wheel, the Falls, the half-moon bridge, and butterfly-tree island. The Tye River connected and streamed steadily down to the valley floor as I followed its S-curves and occasional sudden precipitous dips. Driving on the > right side of the narrow road was risky (a whole new experience of staying between the lines) and I no longer had the rocky cliff face to hug as I did on the way up to my destination. Just a few feet more to the right and I too (like the river) could have dropped off into the gorgeous gorge carved by the river running far below.

As I evened out my drive onto the Tye Valley floor, I took time that one last midday morning to inspect the homes and the ripened fields as I rolled by. The fields were already well past their second harvest and final plantings were lush and ripe. Bales of hay stood lined up at the farthest reaches of some of the properties, signs of separation and dividing lines between the farmers, fields, and forested woods.

Copses of trees often separated homesteads, and some of those in turn were nestled deep into arms of rocky outcroppings. The rising sun shined brightly through my windshield forcing me to put on a pair of sun-glasses and tilt the visor forward. I signaled more short waves to those on the road again, sending especially enthusiastic waves to those who were returning to the hills from the main road. After two days in the hills such as I had had, it was time for me to return back to the main road, to the world-at-large, for I had already taken the road less traveled.

     I stopped off at a tiny Bar-B-Que place for lunch and gave my order, waiting patiently while their specialty was slapped on a bun and heated in the microwave. Back at the motel, I grabbed a diet soda from the machine, chatted with the maids for a while and then huddled myself back into my room to enjoy my feast. Then, I allowed myself the indoor luxury of a short nap, hoping to wake up in time to take my time getting over to Rita and James's home for more talk that afternoon and a homemade dinner with all the trimmings. Like natural clockwork, I woke up exactly at the time I had set.

Part V: Lost Music Refrain

Before the End

I have climbed the mountain only to note that the cycle is not yet complete, nor will it ever be, forever and ever into eternity. I am shaken by this realization and must once more return to the source of creative power of One. My path is indirect now without a goal in mind. Caution and wariness call my steps before the end; curiosity pulls me ever forward in concert with the dance of which I must play my part.

Rita called at the moment I woke up from my afternoon nap. We were to get together for some more talk and an early dinner with James that evening. Each of us was eager to take a break from intense activities of the day. Call it a change in activities for me—settling in for some good solid *human* conversation. It would be good to clear my mind a bit from all of the spacey wanderings of that morning, and those that had risen to critical mass over the previous two days and nights. Time to downshift for a spell, disengage my haunts and musings, and return to ground.

What could I say to anyone at that time anyway? How could I even begin to explain the zap on the mountain (we called each other) where I somehow (magically) stood aligned at the axis between heaven and earth? How too, to explain the playful dance with the butterflies, the flights into past haunts that had somehow been conjured up in the now of then? What words could capture those vivid fluttering (breathing) sounds, the vibrant colors that had (shuffled randomly) scintillated and transported me, the communication that followed no form of communication we humans (normally) understand? I was still in the process of assimilating the whirl of experiences and locating anchor points to tag them for future reference.

      I wanted to re-call them.

  I needed time—a change of pace—in order to digest and integrate all that had happened and delve deeper into the mystery of (why?) my magic mountain area. So, I simply tabled the day's experiences in the back of my mind and let them swirl and sort themselves out in the background.

  Rita and I picked up from our talk the day before with hardly a missed beat. Our happy talk sparked with laughter and release, and continued right on up to dinner preparation when James joined us. What a lot of fun we had! We shared notes about cooking, traveling, ancient cultures, languages, science, bowling, cats, and the flora and fauna (the butterflies!) of the local Blue Hills. My hosts were both so very gracious and I felt like an honored guest. And the meal they planned was literally fit for royalty! James grilled steaks on the barbecue while Rita roasted and rolled small potatoes in light oil sprinkled with her special recipe of rosemary, garlic, salt and pepper, and tossed a fresh garden salad.

  While I helped with the salad fixing, several

cats came into the cheery kitchen to inspect me. One or two at a time, they would come in to patrol the area, take turns to gather handfuls of warm cuddles, and look expectedly at their food dishes. It was feeding time at the zoo for all of us, including an adopted family of raccoons waiting on the back deck. Their comfortable "family" environment and feeding routine making me more than a little homesick for Ed and our own two kitties back home.

I would be driving home the next morning.

After dinner and cleanup we all retired to the back screened-in porch, lit several candles and just recouped from our meal and the day. Yet I could tell that they were anxious to get back to their website work; it would be a long night still ahead for them. On the other hand, I was anxious about driving down their hill and finding my way back to the main road at nighttime. When nightfall descends on the Blue Hills it is exquisitely dark. The moon, who might have been a guiding light, could not guide me that evening—for she had already recessed to her silent sliver stage over the past three nights.

Gracious as ever, Rita and James walked me out to my car. James thoughtfully toted the box of colored pens and design books I had brought to show to them that afternoon. Remarkably, the air smelled especially thick and juicy with moisture. And a slight breeze signaled that perhaps a change was in the air. Together we speculated on the possibility that some soaking thunderstorm might come through the next day. The area desperately needed rain to wash the shrubs and trees, enliven the summer flowers, and feed the Tye River that connected the mountains to harvest valley below.

After hugs all around and making sure that I had clear directions back to the main road, we said our goodbyes. I was to drive down the narrow gravel hill, out from the hilltop, and continue on for a few turns to the main road. I had taken that road several times before in daylight.

But, as it turned out, my day of adventure was not yet over that evening. I took a wrong > right turn right after the hilltop. Not realizing my mistake, I drove merrily on, following the twists and turns of the other road until I could go no farther. The road came to an abrupt dead-end. Suddenly, and only then, I found myself deep in the thicket of Lost.

Lost on the Mountain

It is exceptionally dark in the mountains once the sun goes down. The black dome of sky dips deeply into the overarching canopy of trees and the thicket of woods is all surrounding. No streetlights, no road signs, no sign of human activity anywhere. Driving gives one a limited view from the windows and that only as far as the headlights can penetrate into the dense brush or to seek the road ahead. A sudden wrong turn could have left me spinning into the labyrinth of folding hills or until morning when daybreak would yield some signs of life and I could see where I was going again. Once I realized that I was lost, I tried to retrace my path only to find myself stopped completely at another dead-end.

However, I was lost in a friendly mountain area. I knew that. I had seen it in daylight several times over the 1980s and knew that many of the folks who had moved to the region were just trying to get into a more peaceable way of life, be self-sufficient along the numerous country roads. But by the time I dead-ended, I had no idea where I was. My internal mapping of the area (including the way to Dianne's cabin, the Falls and even back to Rita and James's) was hopelessly mixed up.

What to do? The butterflies, who might have helped navigate me out of my locked position, were asleep. The dome of the night sky was quickly dropping to earth and the woods were closing in on three sides. Because I do not backup well and the road had reduced narrow enough to just fit my car, I saw that I could not turn around. It was the strangest feeling, feeling trapped like that, nose in, and unable to make a move.

The night was incredibly alive, but its secrets well hidden. I tried to lift above the scene get a more panoramic view, but was stopped by some darker than dark hovering "ceiling." It is difficult to explain, but I felt genuine fear for the first time ever in those hills. Even with the door knocks at the Crabtree Falls cabin eleven years before, I had not felt pure fear in the mountains like that.

I felt that I was being watched from above and, remarkably, was being followed. I chided myself: Stay in the car and turn around, find any familiar road, Suzanne. This is all in your mind, Suzanne! You have had a long day full of imaginative adventures here and there, and now you are just on overload.

But I *was* being calm and reasonable about the situation, I replied back to myself. Boy, was I ever reasonable, making all sorts of rational comebacks to my fears. But reasoning didn't help. So I did the most logical thing I could think of in the situation: I maneuvered a full 180 degree, eight point (or more) turn, pulling up and backing out in a tiny tight circle until I could see the road again. Then I started driving slowly and was immensely relieved when the woods backed off from the side of the car. Dust flew around me from the lack of a good rain as dirt and gravel crunched under my wheels. Visibility was so low that I barely ventured a look side to side—my eyes were glued forward. I was determined to backtrack on that dead-end road, so not to get even more lost in the night maze. I would hang in there, creeping forward, until I reached any familiar landmark.

But whatever was above, watching me below, was still there. That was creepy! I could viscerally feel it and it made my skin crawl. The night had been indigo clear, the stars beautiful and twinkling friendly when I had left the Rita and James's home. Now I could not see the sky above but could feel it—something was encroaching downward, a blacker than black ink just above me, blocking out my "view" to the starry cosmos above.

I drove on.
I felt I was being followed.
I tried to pay attention to the road and block out my fear from whatever was observing me from above.
I felt so small, so helpless.
I had to get the hell out of there.
I had my reasons.

Haunting Memory

When I was eight years old and we were still living in Anacortes, life was pretty normal on the island in contrast with what was to come. Mom had given up her day job at the hospital to be with us girls full-time. In addition, in those days, she led a group of Blue Birds, the elementary version of Camp Fire Girls, while Dad worked as first-aid man for the oil refinery, instructed at the local Red Cross, and led a group of Boy Scouts in his off-hours. One night, the refinery called him in for a horrible emergency. There had been an explosion at the plant and several men were burned badly.

(Burns were his specialty and he helped at the hospital.)

With Dad out, Mom and we girls played some games to bide our time as night began to close in around us. It was around eight o'clock when Mom got a call from our next door neighbor
(not Mae's family, the one living on the other side
who coincidentally had the same ethnic last name as my first husband whom I would meet eight years later in high school
on the
other side of the
country)
asking her to bring something—a cup of sugar or flour—for a recipe she was making.

Mom would be right back, she said. While I drew the heavy floor length drapes and closed the shades all around the house (it was a nightly ritual when the sun went down), she put my sleepy two-year-old sister to bed, grabbed that cup of something and was on her way.

I waited.

Do you recall how time can stand still for a young child waiting for her parent to come home? There is that sense of expectancy, a bit of a yearning to have all members in their rightful place. Mom never learned to drive, she couldn't, she said. She had tried, but the coordination of her feet and hands with the rights and lefts left her in tears for the complexity of it all. I learned of one time, before my time, when she tried to drive again and drove the car right up into someone's yard, got out, and simply walked away.

In those early years, we spent many evenings waiting for Dad to come home from work or networking at the local Elks Lodge. These were the 1950s and early 1960s after all, and launching a career for him was anything but routine as he tried his hand over a wide range of possibilities. But for that spring night in 1960, his skills were sorely needed and for the first time I can remember, I was left alone at home at night.

I waited for Mom's cozy comfort to return.
Dad would be out late, he said.
Our young worlds revolve around our parents, regardless of their flaws.
For me, my parents were the best,

        and I often said
      so fervently to my friends,
          just to
        make it clear.

 Although our house was brightly lit inside, all warm and homey, nonetheless I began to gather a strange feeling. By then I was already used to strange feelings (people call it intuition, even sixth sense, these days), but this added another quality—diffused fear—that I was unaccustomed to. There was someone outside of the house! I *knew* it, I could *feel* it, even when I could not peer outside through the black night and the drapes were tightly drawn. Perhaps my mind was working overtime because it was a unique situation. I would grant that. However, that visceral sensing, that body-knowing feeling, is less the feeling of "what if" imagination than it is of somehow being "touched" on an extension of myself.

 In later years I would call this feeling "my radar." And it was on full alert!
Someone was outside and "he" was not friendly. I switched to rational mind, chiding myself for being such a baby. I was proud to be my baby sister's baby-sitter for even a short while and took my responsibility most seriously. But the truth was, I *was* beginning to panic because of *that feeling again* and wondering what to do.

 Thankfully at that moment, Mom came home and walked straight into the living room, all happy smiles. I immediately spilled out my worries to her. Bless her, she didn't discount them. Instead, she knew that my weird feelings and casual comments about strangers had proven valid before—sometimes to my parents' supreme embarrassment. Calm, cool, and collected on the outside, always holding things in on the inside, Mom went into our night's routine and told me it was time to get ready for bed. After I had been sent on my way, and emphatically reiterating to her once more about *still* feeling a presence outside, I lingered in the hallway and heard her make a phone call.

Within a few minutes, she was talking to Dad.
I listened.
Her voice told me that she was scared, a novel experience for me.
I watched.

She put the phone down and sprinted quickly through the kitchen out to the attached garage. I surmised that Dad must have told her to lock the back door—he'd stay on the line. She had already locked the front door immediately upon hearing my fears. She returned to the living room within a couple of minutes and grabbed the phone.

"She was right!" She gasped, catching her breath. "There was a man out there! He must have been hiding behind the incinerator (we burned our trash in the backyard weekly in a tall steel can). He must have been waiting to steal her bike—she left it out again. Oh, Bob, I opened the door and saw him. It was dark and he ran down the alley. It was all quiet, so I just took a peek and there he was. He looked at me and I looked at him and then he ran down the alley."

My mother's voice was trembling, her speech running at a breathy, rapid, disjointed pace. She kept saying over and over that Putty was right and then began all those "wondering-ifs" and pleas for holy forgiveness for leaving her girls home alone.

I learned to trust my radar that night—learned how it felt inside and out. Since then, it has kept me safe in tight spots over the years and allowed me to trust my non-physical extensions when conventional sensory cues are not available or obstructed.

An Aside

    Whatever presence hovered over me that night on the mountain
        higher than the treetops and lower than the starry sky
            (an in-between place)
                remains a
          mystery.

    Eventually, I found my way out of the maze that night. There was a turn I recognized (reversed that time), where the dirt path led to the gravel road past the fenced llama farm. A couple of twists later, I was cruising again, and breathed a sigh of enormous relief when I saw the stop sign marking a right > turn just past the community recycling bins. That downhill turn, in turn, joined me onto a two-way road, winding into the valley below. Soon after, I crossed over one of the many low-lying narrow bridges barely rising above the omnipresent Tye River, and knew I was home free. Within minutes, I had found the highway again.

    There is no satisfying Nancy Drew ending to this mystery of the looming sky. Nor is this a tale of missing time or alien abduction. After spending that expansive, glittering morning alone being so totally aligned, the whole experience with the watching "something" encroaching between the earth and sky continues to present an enigma to me.

    Sometimes there simply are no answers. There are mysteries and there are Mysteries. I have racked my brain over that night, recalling the feeling, the sense of being observed from above, the urgency to stay alert, my radar on full alert. I can still recall in minute detail the events and this too brings me no closer to the truth. Perhaps these things are better off forgotten, unsolved, left to rest in peace and yet...

    Lord help me, that is not the way I am made. Nor was it the way I was brought up, the elder daughter of two scientists. There are questions that beg answers and as I continue to write these notes to you (and me) their moments and memories rise again to interconnect along labyrinths of their own,
    seeking patterns,
        seeking resolution,
            seeking meaning.

    I beg the muse to help me understand. Rational logic and all the scientific knowledge in the world will not help at these times. I find myself questioning the mysteries of my life and realize that I am responsible for my own answers.

    I seek closure, but it evades me.
    I seek factual information, but my parents are long dead.
        (They who seemed to know everything.)

    I ask "why?" at every turn and my answers today exist only in the sense of what I can make of them, and in that sense, I realize that only what is meaningful matters. Like Tantalus I push toward my goal of understanding only to find that each roll of the stone out of the abyss falls back and crushes me ever deeper into the haunts of the unknown. But unlike Tantalus, I have never preferred the direct, brute strength route.

     Have I complicated patterns by trying to make sense of them?
         (I catch their subtle essences everywhere.)
    They lead like butterflies
        weaving and bobbing, dancing and lighting their special glow.
           (Even in the darkest dark of worry and doubt).

Unfurl

Each point a perfect center.
Each beginning a perfect seed.
The truth is already known and yet spends its life unraveling, unfolding

as we too struggle to emerge from our protected cocoon of childhood.

Do we dare to remember that original sweetness

which turns so suddenly to bitter loss?
They say that we spend the second half of our lives returning home,
But what of us who have never left the original sanctuary?

Haunting Memory

Both of my parents were keen on the unseen worlds recently uncovered by science. They were wonderful teachers. Back in the Fidalgo Island days—before my sister was born, when Mom was still working at the lab, and I had yet to see Thunderbird's black eyes staring down on me as I reached to grow up—visits to her lab workplace were not uncommon. Those were thrilling times for me, my only other option being to stay with a neighbor family down the other road during the long day.

My extroverted exuberance for noisy play was often too much for that mother, for she would regularly lock me in a closet for an hour or three just to keep me silent. No one heard my cries from the closet. I tried to explain when I returned home those evenings. Upon my unintelligible pleading, begging for babysitter relief, Mom would give in and take me to her lab, if I promised to be a good girl for her.

And in my best four-year-old manner, I complied.

Her hospital lab was a mysterious place, all white and black with sparkling glass cabinets. The antiseptic smells of that small local hospital greeted us at the door and permeated the very walls. Sadly, within months I would come to associate those "family" smells
—for it saturated our clothes and hair—
with the abject terror of having an ether mask placed over my face.
Count slowly, Dad had said, as he stood by my side in the operating room holding my hand. It was time for

my tonsillectomy. He promised that the excruciating earaches would go away and I, like millions of little kids in those days, was bribed with the promise of unlimited ice cream.

Those horrible earaches—aural defense manifesting in painful, swollen deafness?

What was I hearing that I didn't want to hear?

What angry words spoken I don't seem to remember?

However, in the land of the unseen, Mom was my first teacher. She would help me climb up onto her little metal working stool and first show me a slide with a smear on it. Then, when I determined that it was nothing extraordinary, she would place it under her microscope and have me take a look.

Oh wow! Was there anything more exciting than what I was seeing?

I began pointing to the slide, questioning my line of sight (before and after, above and below), and then would take another look back down the black tubes into the world of the microscope.

It was a whole new world! There were critters swimming and floating, rushing and colliding and squiggling everywhere that I could see.

Mom called them "tiny animals" and told me that they were everywhere—in the ponds with the frogs, in the raindrops, the grass—we just didn't see them with our unaided eyes. We live in an amazing world, she said, there are things that we do not see, but with science's help we can.

I was sold!

>Science was the word.

>And from that day forward, the unseen could be just as "real" as the seen world. I learned that it was only a matter of (infinite) perspective and the (tuning) instruments available to the observer.

Over my early years, I would be told about all sorts of unseen worlds described in exquisite detail via chalk talks delivered by Dad. He was a frustrated professor, I am convinced of that, and there was always a story behind the story taught in school.

"Did I want to know?" or "Did I *really* want to know?" He would ask just as soon as I asked a question that would catch his fancy—and I could discern whether or not he was in a "good mood." Those were some of the best of times in my childhood growing into my teen years, when the emotional climate surrounding us would suddenly swing calm for just a few hours and I could sense enough harmony among us to ask a question. One very special talk I recall so well was the one about the electromagnetic spectrum. Having spent his days in Anacortes running the x-ray lab and manning a shortwave radio, Dad was "the expert" when it came to unseen waves of all sorts. During one definitive lecture I will never forget, he taught me about some of the unknown properties, the hidden gaps, in the electromagnetic spectrum.

Dad called them cosmic rays—if I recall correctly.

He said that they might be where the "psychic stuff" occurred.   Curious, because the science teachers at school didn't talk of more than three time dimensions, I had asked the physics teacher about more than four,

                              and received zero.

Speculations of the unknown, delving into mysteries of the Universe,
                      science revealed no answers.
                If science was the word in my childhood,
        then science lessons in school bombed, imploded
                      into rattling rote answers divinely flat, lifeless, and rigid.

I wanted answers.

I am still seeking answers in this Nancy Drew world of hidden clues. Mysteries infinitely greater than the place where answers seem to lie, for those answers live beyond thresholds I have not yet crossed. But in that late summer of 1998, on those mountains of the Blue Hills, windows of the sky flashed open and the magic returned.
The patterns of Life,
        all things my parents tried to share with
    me—

about their love of worlds
unseen, unknown,
so joyously they endeavored to convey to be
flashed in illumination that day in
synchrony—
no longer divided by splintered
fragments of self and time.

Unfurl

*Is there anyone so wretched as my mother
       who would choose to escape into the
unknown before her time?*

*What piercing anguish must have turned to a
cancer over her years
       (suffering shades of soulless black,
           hearing dirges in silent
       desperation)
I cannot fathom its darkness for its depths!*

*Where was the light, my dear mother,
       and why was yours so cruelly
extinguished?*

*I do not blame you—I want to understand you.
           You, who were always so
         innocent and gentle;
                 full of the dreams of life
                 in joyous exploration of
             the seen and the unseen
         (whether or not it was sensory sight that
you were sharing)
              in my earliest years.*

After the End

I have concluded my progress and still have not met my elusive goal—it does not exist except in the realm of confusion after the end. I have reached a place of perfect equilibrium and to go further will only disrupt the balance of forces attained along my way. And yet, I must take the next step to see what lies ahead; taking note of what has gone before me as the cycle moves to my less than rapture.

My third day in the Blue Hills heralded a repeat of the previous two. An early morning promise of sultry hot arose hours before the sun had a chance to suck the morning dew out of the night's barely dampened fields. The much needed rain had not been forthcoming, so I extended myself in empathy out to the wilted wildflowers, crackled shrubbery, and faded woodland grasses for their unrelenting plight. It was difficult to imagine that once in the not so distant past the Tye River had topped its mountain gorges, overflowed its banks, and flooded the whole valley below.

Such are the cycles within cycles of Nature—no different from those of my own. The mountain had called me to her and already it was my time to leave her embrace again. I paid my bill as soon as the office opened and took one last walk out into the field behind the little motel. All of nature was reanimating once more, busy to get on with the tasks of the day before the sun rose high in the sky and cool shelter would be difficult to find. Off to the far > side I followed a little wooded path, listening to the bustle of birds as they fearlessly crisscrossed and darted overhead. I reflected on the night before, about being lost in the

Blue Hills. My feelings then—they had been so real! What a swarm of stinging memories helpless dread had buzzed up! Now in the early morning daylight again with the birds singing from all quarters and after a good night's sleep, I could only laugh at myself.

       Silly, indeed! I had lived up to my nickname once again.

Haunting Memory

It was the night of my 38th birthday. By comparison, deep winter is relatively easy in Richmond, Virginia. If there had been an icy snow, more likely than not it would drop like a smothering blanket during that week. I had learned by experience that particular probability over my nine years

> (and seven homes
> each with a climate of its own
> —I am my father's daughter,
> after all)

in that rapidly growing city. But there had been no snow that week and I looked forward the next morning to redecorating the downstairs half bath of my new fifteen-year-old condominium.

I sat on the edge of the bed in the dark. It was already in the wee hours approaching my birth time and date. I had a lot to be grateful for in 1990 to tell my parents. I began talking to them in my mind, thanking them for the person I had become, thanking them for all of their trials and sacrifices to raise me the best way that they knew how.

> (They were young after all.)

I empathized and reached out to them with all of my heart, returning to the better, earlier times and lessons their short lives had shared with me. I reflected.

The last time I had seen my mother alive she was also 38—well past her point of no return. Dad's death left her spiraling down to ever blacker days over the next eight and a half years, the last three spent as a quadriplegic. Whether she jumped or fell or was pushed out of her second story window we never knew. She landed on her back, all broken, pierced, and ruptured. She pleaded with me on the phone a few days before her death, imploring me to understand that she did not jump. I believe her.

My father died suddenly at 42, two weeks after my high school graduation, after efforts to reconstruct his colon failed. He kept his prophetic promise to me and made medical history as the longest living survivor of a rare congenital defect.

I reflected upon them with all the love within me. Without warning, the dark room (and my open heart) was filled with the greatest rush of pure love! Amidst the tiny blue sparkles once again dancing around me,

>I felt an overwhelming compassion returning
>>back to me,
>>>surrounding me,
>>>>soothing me,
>>>>>celebrating with

me.
>My face and hair were stroked with affection.
>>(It was a most awesome

communion of spirit.)

Sometimes when we are lucky, in-tune, and aligned just so, life throws us an additional morsel of synchronistic validation to let us know that our insights and intuitions, our feelings and connections, are right on. I *knew* in my heart of hearts that night that my parents were once again with me, permeating every cell of the room and my soul. Similar to connecting glow beams with the butterflies, we had created our own unique form of communication where there was no separation of start and stop, them and me, life and death; just one continuous flow of Being in resonance through the very core of Us.

    The synchronistic morsel came the next day, still on my birthday.

On the plasterboard wall, under three or four layers of old wallpaper I steamed and scraped off that day,
    in the half bath of my condo,
        two-thousand miles from where I spent my early Fidalgo years,
            was my nickname written by a long gone construction worker
                was a single note in ink:
                    "Putty."

Artist Musings

When I think of life as one huge canvas
    upon which the brush strokes of
experience are drawn,
        where, when, and how do the
        colors, textures and patterns
            begin to emerge?
When do I step back and observe the picture as a whole,
    and when do I need to walk up close,
        stick my very eyes (i's) into the
    fine pointillist detail
            (only to lose sight of the
            overall impressions of the
            painting before me)?

And when do I finally, simply, take a deep breath, walk into the canvas,
    to become my own expression of
forever living art?

Haunting Memory

Because Mom didn't drive and in our later years as a family, Dad would often spend hours lying prone on the couch in front of the TV on weekends and after work, my sister and I were left to our own devices. The home climate became increasingly touchy, we never knew what the next wave of suicidal depression or sudden explosive rage would bring.

It was better to walk on eggshells and try to become invisible.

That was easier for me to do, especially during and after the Death Valley days when I could disappear for hours with my friends and enjoy walking outside with them, covering wide distances, just talking "normally" about school and boys, orchestra and clubs.

Above all topics, the family secrets must remain secret.
It was the unsaid rule of the household.
I didn't dare compromise it.

I so enjoyed strolling alone out in the open desert sand and scrub, and years later walking through the deep woods along the creek that ran about a quarter mile behind our duplex in Arlington. Hours spent alone just walking, thinking, trying to figure out how to best to approach my parents for this or that, anticipating their reactions and trying to circumvent any more grief.

I was lucky—I could get out and walk. I had school friends I could visit.

My sister had none of these during our short twelve years living together as a family. She was clumsy in her stride and didn't walk far. She would fall or fall behind when playing with others, and more often than not, she would retreat to her room, quiet as a mouse so as not to upset the house. She didn't want to get caught in the crossfire and was precociously sensitive to the vibes around her.

Amazing how similar walking on eggshells is to toeing the Indian Walk
   (so as not to disturb the natural world around us).

(My sister's mild cerebral palsy and seizures would not be medically validated for another twenty to thirty years. This proclamation caused her former orchestra conductor to exclaim that her skill with the violin in the face of CP was no less the feat of an one-legged skier winning the Olympics.

I'll never forget that joy of discovery and accomplishment in her voice when she first told me what he had said. She had been through so much over her young life. The diagnosis answered many frustrating questions that had confronted her.)

So many childhood mysteries left untapped, nameless
    —denial buried deeply in our family house of secrets.
        The sanctuary had gone haywire.

An Aside

The rule of the house was unspoken but well understood: What goes on in our family is our own business; do not tell a soul. This meant not talking to well-meaning teachers.

("Does your husband beat your daughter, Mrs. Brown? She seems very intimidated around me." My seventh grade math teacher was tall and strong, sported a crew cut and black-rimmed glasses like my dad. How could he know the resemblance?

"Oh no," Mom replied, "Suzanne is the pride of his eye." Her own eyes downcast, voice already slightly slurred that morning. That parent-teacher meeting was one of her last ventures out before she began to hide in the house all day).

And there were several who took an active interest in my zeal for scholarship, languages and the violin. I remember them fondly—their encouraging words and acts of kindness over those hellish years—relief and sustenance for this little girl.

I was stuck. Home became a prison for me while it was a sanctuary for them. We had strict rules for my friends, too—when they could visit (only with prior notice) and when they could phone (not when anyone was sleeping, which was often). Not a few times when a friend dropped by, Dad would answer the door dressed in his robe and blow the kid away with angry words about impertinence, no proper respect for his daughter.

    Dad was fiercely protective of his domain.
    Yet he would bellow and call me a whore (that stung me to tears) when I first began to wear makeup. Master Bobby's ideal of the Southern Lady sprung from his own gentrified childhood, which included a household of servants, academy schooling, and debutante balls. His anger with his father for "disowning" him after Dad quit pre-med (after WWII had drafted and disillusioned him) glowered always just a little bit under the surface. We, the children, inherited the incessant criticism Dad's own father held over him.

            There are many forms of abuse.
    For me, it was never knowing from one day to the next what the emotional weather highs and lows would bring. I had to deal with it. I had no choice.
        I had learned how to test the waters
           imperceptibly
                  —to keep on my toes and dance
            lightly.
             I was ever vigilant.

When I graduated from high school, I could leave. I yearned for the day.
    All I wanted was to escape. But how could I, in the realm of possibilities?
        Then the Sister Fates took that weighty decision away from me.

Unfurl

Oh gentle and passionate parents, you who were so full of Life!
I knew you when you still had spirit in your eyes and life and its bitter passage had not dulled nor tarnished
your luster, your beauty, your hope.

How could everything have gone so wrong?
When exactly did your hopelessness begin?
I silently observed your transition, sinking deeper into despair
—once laughing butterflies of exquisite promise, genius, and creativity transformed to empty ashy husks of cocoons—
(a reverse evolution)
and I was helpless to shift the course of that river.

You were my gods; you knew all the answers, you could do anything!
Then you left me to make all of the decisions for you.
I couldn't, I couldn't, I couldn't.

Haunting Memory

During the last years in our Arlington home, Mom would plead, shake and beg for my help. Dad would withdraw to the couch in front of the TV or sleep on his days off work to forget. Sometimes, when the climate shifted calm all around, Dad and I would get into an engrossing game of chess, or Mom and I would enjoy preparing meals, discussing classical music and books. Then, during those times, my sister would venture out of her room, sensing all was safe, and for a while we would all play silly games and laugh together as a family again. It was great for both of us to see Mom and Dad hug, telling us how much they loved each other and us girls.

It was so confusing! Rarely was there a stormy silence. Punishment for us girls was simple—and heavy enough when we were put "in the dog house"— Dad's form of shunning us until he felt like we understood a point he was making. More often than not *the point* was one of caviler criticism, depending more on his moods than our actions. The climate of perpetually being on guard as a child (lightly toeing the Indian walk so as not to disturb Nature around us) was simply miserable. Psychologists today call this a "double bind." That is, being told one thing (you can be anything you want to be, you have it all), but these particular things, do not do or talk about (for they upset the equilibrium of our sanctuary, our secret place).

Round and round in circles we went, the cycles spinning ever tighter inside the house, inside ourselves, where the homesickness seemed, by those seams, to have no way out for any of us.

So it was a great relief that on one day there was great excitement, a breath of hope was in the air. Dad had drawn a little figure on the chalkboard. Mom and Dad hugged and giggled like teenagers. With a flourish of a grand announcement they pointed to the chalk figure and said that it was an illustration of baby Brown—a new sister or brother was in the making! Oh! You should have seen their faces light up, the spirit sparkle return to their eyes for those few days waiting for the rabbit to die.

>
> (What in the hell were they thinking?)
> But the rabbit didn't die.
>> Life returned to "normal" for three more months.
>>> Then, on that July 4th weekend, those spirals collided, imploded.
>> Unexpectedly, Death gave Dad his predicted out,
>>> and family life as I knew it
>>> abruptly ended.

An Aside

How did I get so off track from the enchantment of this Blue Hills Diary? My magic mountain area had called me and I had responded. We performed our dance in perfect synchrony. It is an enigma to me that such a transformative experience of bliss and light should be so shrouded in the shadowy residue of heavy haunts of bygone days.

It has been two years since I began writing these notes to you and me. What wrenching sorrow reignited on the mountain to unfold during the course of these writings! Creeping shadows awakened out of their slumber. What hells burst through dammed rivers of emotions carved deep within the gorges of my psyche! Had the rivers and gorges been there all along, merely covered over in later years by the flotsam and debris of an otherwise normal everyday life? In my artist's walk along the road of beauty and majesty in life, did I forget the ugly, the painful—those early years glossed and lost to feeling for four decades?

No, it simply was my time to remember;
    to view life's tapestry backwards,
forward, and inside out.
    This was the gift of the Blue Hills.

Epilogue

It is time to return to the whole of me that is more than the fragments of my recollections. There are, of course, many fragments not entered into this diary. Yet there is a hidden magic that seeks to meld all experience in every life—"magic" in this case meaning that which we do not yet know or understand. The mystery remains. We ask again the question: Who am I? That question begs for more. More than circular intellectual debates testing the prevailing winds of the nature-nurture controversy which seem to forever rage on the battlefields of academe. The "Who am I?" question is powerfully, intimately personal, and one I feel necessary before any claims can be made of knowing truth, solving grand mysteries. What hubris it is when we claim to know all and yet have not even begun to know our self!

In a larger sense each one of us must eventually come to our own findings, insights, truths, where we no longer rest in the comfort of absolutes and dogmas that have been shaping and strapping human consciousness for eons. At times of great perplexities and wrenching losses we are forced to reach deeper into our souls, in search to discover that which lives unseen beyond our human manifestation and collective perceptions.

To dare not is living death! For then we remain merely the husk of a desiccated cocoon of unrealized and trapped human potential—where life's promise sleeps still unbidden beneath the surface, never breaking free of those confines that continue to imprison and haunt us. To carry the banner of another's paradigm or philosophy, be it church, state, or science, reduces us to mere robots. For in that guise we go through the motions of the day to day. Yet, sooner or later, the droning of the communal hive leaves us unnourished, starving, parched for what we know not in recent memory. A longing for something long since forgotten, and yet haunting hints of *that* something we never lost.

The story of the Blue Hills Diary is one of personal renewal and resurrection—a book begun with the overwhelming joy of homecoming that led to a rebirth discovered, born out of ashes of grief and loss. I did not know this when I began to write this story of mystical transcendence. Although I was called to journey back that particular place and time—there and then, where and when in a few precious moments, my whole life flashed before me—it has taken me at least two years to even begin to integrate, gestate, and birth the magnificence of it all. What holy union of earth and sky stunned, zapped, and infused me? What sacred conception within changed the past of dull lead into the rich gold of now to unfold, birth in its own sweet time of return?

The butterflies taught me about relative time, that language is spoken without words. Their message is to discover our common empathy that moves deeper than surface expectations. The mountains reminded me of what is everlasting and always, for these times of "tie me" only begin with initial awareness of understanding. Only then do we stand under what we catch, what is thrown our way across times forgotten, those out of time times that lives between the here and there.

There were many renderings of those moments

that beg for expression. At times, pure awe and wonderment carried me gently on waves of soft golden morning light, floating on warm river drafts, rising upward to dance above and behold the valley hills that were fulfilling their perennial ripening cycle of life below. I became butterfly and joined them in their playful nets of frolic and frisk. My locus of Self was beyond me. I became a pillar of light stretching into the farthest reaches of outer space and the deepest core of Mother Earth. My locus of Self was within me. For I, like the trees, the rocks and the river, served as a connector and a conduit of all forms of energy imaginable and wept to know that my presence at each and every moment was absolutely necessary, essential, indeed integral to the creation of that moment.

And yet what about the moments in between? Those spaces and times where and when we have the power to create that which is still unformed? Out of the immense sea of void and chaos we catch a flutter, gather a glimpse, hear a sigh, sense a heart. How subtly they stroke the fabric of our life's interconnecting ever-present web! From all dimensions they impinge upon us and in our narrow perceptions we can do no more than represent them as past, present, and future, or deliberate distances structured in terms of space and relative measure. But in every moment there exists an expectancy ready for the Creator's breath of life. For it is in those standstill still-point moments in between the rhythms of breath that we begin life anew, drawing on worlds of possibilities, potential not yet wholly created or destroyed.

The Blue Hills called me and I had answered their call. It was the most extraordinary feeling—a magnetic pull so strong that I could no longer deny it, for it just got stronger, building more insistent over the days prior to my vacation. Something out there was in need. I felt it within my whole being. I learned on my morning hike up to the lower circuit of the Falls that indeed my very breath, sweat and footsteps were necessary to nurture and shape that beautiful mountainscape where thousands before me over the centuries had already viewed, touched and trudged before me. I recognized to my depths my connection with this land, my footsteps before, the former occasions when somehow in some way, magic happened. It was like the Blue Hills themselves caught me in their web on each visitation—each full of enchantment, full of mystery, a call from beyond. Amazing, too, because I had spent my earliest years on the opposite coast of America. It boggles my mind to think of all of the twists and turns my life took that lead to those moments of perfect contentment, a feeling of correctness, knowing that my presence was bidden and absolutely essential. Serendipity is powerful stuff.

Something out there was in need. But I did not know at the time that it was me! The rocks and trees and river and butterflies did a magnificent job mesmerizing me into thinking that they needed me during the duration of my visit, when all along it was I who so sorely needed them—to be healed by them, to be held by them. Like ripples on the water that are sent forth from a central point of time and space, I am still feeling the repercussions of those days in the Blue Hills. On the surface, the enchantment surrounded me in a deep mist of forgetfulness of everything except the pure moment. Only the infusion of Knowledge mattered, and as with most experiences of spontaneous ecstatic enlightenment, I felt connected, united, integral to the great Oneness that we all are. I was fully present in the moment and paradoxically in all times and places. And during those times I was no one and everyone, no thing and everything, and realized in a flash that this was the status quo, whether I was intimately aware of it or not.

     I have had these mystical experiences here and again in my life and they often come just in the time of need, when longing for reassurance of something greater than sleepwalking throughout my day to day deliberations. But even below the surface of enchantment, wonder and awe, ecstasy, bliss and glow beams, there are deeper waters and channels that transport and connect us. It is there, in the deep underground connective channels of unfettered subconsciousness, where we are sparked alive and align with Creation, and we discover the seeds, potential, and promise that have been lying dormant within ourselves all along. We hear our call. Yet mine was not a whisper; it was a shout. In a perfect reciprocal uroborous circle of need and fulfillment, the hills and my psyche received what we each needed from the other those days. Yet we were not divided. And like ripples that ride on the eternal waters of flowing consciousness that cannot be separated, we continue to benefit in tandem from our fortunate interaction. There is much to say about being at the right place at the right time, but when we begin to see that every place and time is sublime in its correctness, well then, we begin to see our own life themes in full artistic relief. In hindsight, there is a wonderful, unique pattern to it all that has been present all along, just waiting to be embraced, integrated, and fully lived out.

While philosophers and mystics may wax ecstatic about the Journey "Home" with all of its enlightenment and transcendental bliss, they are negligent in not telling us that the Journey "back" after these extraordinary experiences may be fraught with uncertainties, doubts and frustrations.

Over the years I have often talked and shared correspondence with others who have had the pleasure of one or more transcendental mystical experiences. Regardless of the place, time, age and trigger, we discover at core that we are experiencing the grand perennial Knowing that we are connected, not as parts or fragments, but as integral wholly conscious Beings who transcend eons, location and circumstance. Admittedly, this is pretty heady stuff, and for many that is the end of it. Certainly for me on my drive home from the Blue Hills that morning in September (as well as after the 1987 Medicine Wheel days), I felt supremely blessed, with each turn on the road showering me with rainbow rays of sunshine, a sense of anticipation and a brilliance of perception that was simply not of this world.

When I returned home, I wanted more than anything to recapture the feeling, the beauty, the awesome insights that had been my gift to receive. For the first time in my life, I knew what an artist, composer, or poet must feel, driven to capture that which is beyond words and larger than circumscribed life. There was an exquisite ache begging for expression that would not let go. Parallel and similar to being called to the Blue Hills, I could not deny it. Universe then upped the ante, and I felt called again, this time to discover some way to express all of the holographic wonder still roiling within me.

The easy part might be telling the story as a linear sequence of events, but this was nothing like that. It was nonlinear, non-rational—a whole ball of shifting angles of impression, feeling, music and dance. I could capture a freeze-frame, similar to the way a painter creates a still-life, snapshot-of-reality picture. But I was not visiting that realm of reality, certainly not what is commonly understood by our culture as "reality." And above all, I took my life-theme infusion that I am a communicator seriously. For in that Knowing, the threads of my life no longer seemed random and chaotic, but clearly there was a pattern to it all—and all (!) I had to do was step backwards and within myself for a spell in order to grasp the magical more that is greater than the sum of its parts. For no doubt, this was the key to salving my ache for creative expression and moving forward in my life again: backward, forward and inside out.

I did not understand that at first. Hindsight is a wonderful thing, particularly when coupled with introspection.

But how to express these numinous, ineffable experiences that are more than the immediate wonder of the moment? How do we catch a rainbow of mermaids that sings to us? A butterfly who dances her whole life cycle before us? An anchoring rock that recalls us back into the untapped depths carved by childhood pain? Oh my dears, how do we capture, with whole heart and soul, those infinite reverberations of otherworldly color, music, and dance that course through the cosmos and within every cell of our bodies? And when we have met face to face with our whole life recall in a blissfully vibrant call-to-life *mandate to bring it back home*—how do we transform that ache to create, to *communicate* this knowledge into something abiding, living beyond a still-life reproduction and linear sequences of words?

    I let the Muse lead. I had no option, for I was at a loss as to how to even begin beyond waxing ecstatic about the whole business. I had to trust that which had been infused, even though at the time I had no clue about what all had been set in motion, planted in those days. I certainly had no conscious knowledge of the course it would take and whether it would ever take root, germinate, spring forth and unfold—or die on the vine. Many times in the early days of writing, I argued with the Muse. But she would not let go—and in truth neither could I—for I had received my mandate to communicate these experiences in the Blue Hills and before I knew it, the Muse led me deeper and deeper into the rich, untapped ores of my earth, my center, my Self and my pain. And my healing. For truly, the Blue Hills had more in store for me those days than just a pleasant walk in the park.

    The result is this *Blue Hills Diary*. It was born out of a labor of love.

September 2000

CPSIA information can be obtained at www.ICGtesting.com
Printed in the USA
LVOW042025111012

302424LV00001B/20/P